Helen Ken... ... 2012
Cognitive T... 012
Mental Healt... ... in the treatment
of anxiety and childhood trauma. She has made valuable
contributions to the field of Cognitive Behavioural Therapy
through her workshops and writings, which include the bestselling
Overcoming Anxiety, as well as *An Introduction to Cognitive
Behaviour Therapy*. She is the director of the Oxford Advanced
Cognitive Therapies Studies course and in 2002 she was voted one
of the most influential female Cognitive Behavioural Therapists in
Britain by members of the British Association for Behavioural and
Cognitive Psychotherapies.

C015147875

Also by Helen Kennerley

Overcoming Anxiety
Managing Anxiety: A Training Manual
An Introduction to Cognitive Behaviour Therapy (co-author)
An Introduction to Coping with Childhood Trauma
Overcoming Childhood Trauma
Surviving as a CBT Therapist (co-author)

HOW TO BEAT YOUR FEARS AND WORRIES

Helen Kennerley

ROBINSON

Constable & Robinson Ltd
3 The Lanchesters
162 Fulham Palace Road
London W6 9ER
www.constablerobinson.com

First published in the UK by Robinson,
an imprint of Constable & Robinson Ltd., 2011

Copyright © Helen Kennerley 2011

The right of Helen Kennerley to be identified as the author of this
work has been asserted by her in accordance with the
Copyright, Designs and Patents Act 1988

All rights reserved. This book is sold subject to the condition
that it shall not, by way of trade or otherwise, be lent, re-sold,
hired out or otherwise circulated in any form of binding or cover
other than that in which it is published and without a similar condition
including this condition being imposed on the subsequent purchaser.

A copy of the British Library Cataloguing in
Publication Data is available from the British Library

Important
This book is not intended as a substitute for advice or medical treatment.
Any person with a condition requiring medical attention should consult
a qualified medical practitioner or suitable therapist.

ISBN 978-1-84901-399-4

Printed and bound in the EU

1 3 5 7 9 10 8 6 4 2

ACKNOWLEDGEMENTS

Therapists can only write these sorts of books because of the insights that their patients give them and so I'm grateful to those people I've been fortunate enough to help over the years. I'm also particularly grateful to Michele Kirsch, who has done her best to make this a more readable text, so that more of you might be able to benefit from it.

CONTENTS

WHAT YOU NEED TO KNOW BEFORE READING THIS BOOK

Fear, stress, worry and anxiety. These are all common terms for feelings that can cause problems and really interfere with our quality of life. This book will show you ways of managing them – it will give you some basic coping skills. These skills are not a 'cure' but ways to reduce the impact anxieties and fears have on your life. Although 'fear', 'stress', 'worry' and 'anxiety' are slightly different from each other, in this book the terms will be used as if they are similar and the strategies you will learn can help you get on top of them.

In order to get the most out of any self-help book, you'll need to do more than just read through it – you'll need to do the exercises *and* practise the skills you learn. After all, if you bought a diet book but didn't follow the diet, you wouldn't lose weight. However, if you do read this book and follow the exercises you will gain a better understanding of your anxieties *and* you will learn some basic coping skills, which will help you reduce the problems they cause.

This self-help approach, based on the principles of Cognitive Behavioural Therapy (CBT), aims to put you back in control of your own thoughts, feelings and behaviour, so that you do not feel overwhelmed or restricted by worries and fears. You may be familiar with some of the techniques and you might even have tried them before. If they didn't work for you the first time, don't give up! It doesn't mean that you failed, or that the techniques are not right for you. It's possible you weren't in the right frame of mind to fully engage in the work (and it is work), or perhaps you didn't give it enough time, or were too harsh on yourself. Interestingly, there is good evidence that not being harsh or unforgiving to yourself in the course of CBT practice will help it work for you.

HOW TO ADOPT A COMPASSIONATE ATTITUDE

In CBT, it has always been important to practise self-talk – the conversation you have with yourselves in your head – to encourage yourself to try out new ways of behaving and new ways of seeing things. It has become clear in recent years that the WAY you talk to yourself is also important. So if your inner voice is a bit of a bully, and you beat yourself up for not completing a task, or use negative language to spur yourself into doing something ('Come on, you idiot, get on that plane right now or you will ruin everything and let the family down.'), it is less likely that you will get the result you need. In order to make CBT really work, you have to be *compassionate* to yourself, and use gentle, encouraging language, as you would with someone you cared about. There will be plenty of examples of this in the book to help get a feel for the compassionate attitude, and you can read more about being compassionate in Professor Paul Gilbert's book, *The Compassionate Mind* (see 'Useful Books and Resources' at the end of this book).

So, if you find an exercise challenging or difficult, be gentle and encouraging to yourself no matter what the outcome. For example, if you have a fear of going to the cinema or a restaurant, a compassionate approach would be to recognize that this is difficult and to give yourself permission to build up to the challenge in small steps, perhaps taking along a supportive friend with you and certainly using the techniques you will learn in this book to manage your anxiety levels. If the outing is not a success, a compassionate approach would be to give yourself a pat on the back for trying, and then try again, or take a step back and try something else still challenging but less difficult. The non-compassionate approach would be to push yourself too far too soon and then criticize yourself for not meeting the challenge or, if you did meet the challenge, downgrading your achievements: 'That was no big deal, everyone can go to the cinema.' Do you recognize any of these non-compassionate responses?

It's also important to remember that there's a big difference between self-compassion and opting for trying to avoid the problem – you'll need to get the balance right. Later in this book, we'll discuss avoidance in more detail so that you'll be better at recognizing it. There will be times when you're just not able to face your fear and it's OK to accept this when it happens, but overcoming your anxieties will mean eventually facing the uncomfortable feelings that arise when you try something new. Telling yourself, 'I won't go the cinema, or restaurant, because it's just too difficult and I'll feel anxious, like I always do,' is more akin to avoidance than compassion. But more about that later.

As you can see, your attitude towards yourself is important. In this book you'll read about several ways in which anxieties can show themselves and the names given to these different types. These labels are helpful to an extent, but it's crucial to not get hung up on them and VERY important not to think of yourself only in terms of your diagnosis. So, you are not 'a phobic', or 'an agoraphobic' – instead, you are a person who has problems with anxiety, or a person who has a phobia and, most importantly, a person who might also have a meaningful job, a family, a nice personality, a great sense of humour, and so on. Again, it's about attitude. If you define yourself by your problem and you're not compassionate towards yourself, you limit your awareness of your strengths. You can also risk giving an unfair impression of yourself and others might make assumptions about you which are not true. Your anxiety is a *part* of you, but it is not *you*. With the help of this book you can begin to develop a more positive outlook and a better idea of who you are, so you'll be able to be confident that you can do more of the things you want to do and be more the person that you want to be.

GETTING READY

You've bought the book and you're ready to go – it's tempting to turn straight to the coping strategies and 'top tips' for change. But your success will depend on good groundwork – you need to be able to make the ideas in this book work for *you*, and that rests on you getting a good understanding of *your* difficulties – so that you can make your coping plan *personal*. Therefore, the first half of this book goes into a lot of detail about anxieties, fears, worries and stress in order to help you pinpoint what drives your problems. When you have a good idea of this, you can build up the right coping plan for *you* which will be based on your sound understanding of *your* fears and worries.

The second half of the book introduces you to a wide range of coping strategies that you can choose from. You'll learn about controlled breathing and how to relax to ease physical discomfort; thought management to tackle worrying thoughts; graded practice and problem-solving to help you face your fears; and you'll learn how to cope in the long term – how to make coping part of your life.

When you start to face your fears, you'll do best if you have a familiar collection or range of coping methods. This means that you'll need to practise the techniques in this book so that you know them well and have confidence in them. They also need to be well rehearsed enough for you to be able to call on them as you need to – even in times of stress.

It is probably a good idea to first read the whole book through before starting your 'programme' – just to get familiar with anxiety disorders, the CBT approach and to get a sense of how it can help you. You can then work through the actual techniques in the book, taking one section at a time and trying to master one strategy before you move on to the next step. If you try something for a good while and find your anxiety levels are not coming down, don't worry, simply move on. You can always come back to the earlier section when you're ready. Not every technique will work for everyone, but do try each one so that you give yourself the best chance of developing the widest range of coping strategies possible for you. It's difficult to say just how long you should try any one method, but certainly daily practice for several weeks is a good idea. If you're still not getting results, you might need more time, or more external support from a friend or a professional such as your family doctor.

Once you're familiar with the way this book works and the skills you'll need to manage your fears and worries, you can revisit the chapters that are particularly relevant to you and you can tailor and 'fine-tune' your coping plans to best meet *your* needs.

YOU ARE NOT ALONE

If you read through some of the suggestions and think, 'Oh, I could never do that alone,' then enlist the help of friends and family. If you ask for help, encourage your supporters to read this book, too, so they have a better understanding of your problems and what needs to be done to help you overcome them. It can be difficult to explain your fears and worries to someone who has little or no personal experience of them and this book will give them a basic understanding.

For those of you with more complex anxiety problems, who feel overwhelmed or that you're slipping into depression, it's important to seek professional help in the form of therapy and, in some cases, medication. If you explain your problem to your doctor, he or she will have a variety of counselling and/or medicinal options, depending on the severity of your problem. Do this sooner rather than later. Often people find that with a bit of extra support, they can still follow the methods in this book.

Another effective way to use this book is alongside a CBT therapist who specializes in anxiety and stress. Your therapist will be guided by the same ideas that are in the book and you will have your own reference book to consult between sessions with your therapist.

Although the case illustrations in this book are based on the experiences of people who have struggled with anxiety, none of the cases represent actual people.

1

THE STRESS RESPONSE

Just about everyone will feel stressed, worried, afraid or anxious some of the time. It's normal and, as you'll see later, extremely helpful in most circumstances.

Just like you, many people have fears and worries that cause them problems, although the types of anxieties differ from person to person. Appearances can be deceptive – fears and worries are not always obvious to an outsider – so don't assume that others don't share your difficulties just because you can't see them.

For example, you might see a seemingly confident woman at a party, surrounded by friends and reeling off amusing anecdotes, but in two days' time this woman has to give a small presentation at work and she's dreading it. She's terrified that she will dry up, even though in her social life, she is the life and soul of the party. If she were to admit this fear to a friend at the party, the friend would probably say, 'You? Afraid? No chance!' You might notice a man enjoying taking his children on fairground rides, loving the adrenaline rush almost as much as his kids. What you can't see is that he pales at the thought of a flight to Spain. He knows the fairground ride will last a few minutes, but the flight will be about two hours. And he can't explain his problem because he is not afraid of flying. He just can't stand the thought of being stuck on a plane for that length of time, with no escape.

So it's important to remember that you are not alone or odd in any way because you have difficulties managing some of your fears.

HELPFUL STRESS

Marie and her family were out enjoying a meal in an Italian restaurant.

> *We were very relaxed and enjoying our meal in one of our favourite family restaurants. My husband made a joke and we all started to laugh, but then I noticed my teenage son wasn't laughing. He couldn't seem to catch his breath, and he was turning purple. He pointed to a bowl of olives and I soon understood that he was choking on one that had gone down the wrong way. My heart started to pound, I was shaking slightly and breathing fast. It felt as if the food I'd just swallowed was stuck in my throat, but I immediately jumped up from my seat and grabbed my son from behind and used a manoeuvre I'd been taught a long time ago in first-aid training. After the second try, the olive flew out of his mouth. I felt like crying from relief! After a few minutes and a glass of water, he was fine, but I still felt shaky. My husband told me later that everyone was looking at our table, but I wasn't aware of anything except getting that olive*

out of my son's windpipe. There really wasn't time to think what it looked like. All that mattered was clearing his airway. It was hard for me to enjoy the rest of the meal, but my son was fine. He thought it was funny, the way the olive flew out. Once he laughed I knew he was OK and I was able to relax a bit more.

In this situation, fear helped Marie save her son. Acting on it was absolutely the only thing to do. The fear triggered a rush of adrenaline which prepared Marie to take rapid action to save her son from choking. She was focused only on him, she had only one line of thought (to save him) and she had a burst of energy which gave her the stamina she needed. Afterwards she felt jittery and emotional, which is perfectly normal after any situation involving real danger, and the feeling passed once she knew that her son was safe.

Whenever we read stories in the press about heroic actions or people putting themselves in danger to save others, they always say it was 'automatic' or 'I didn't think about it, I just did it.' That's the stress response in action and it can work very well for us.

In short, this response is helpful, vital even, so we would never want to be without it but we need to be able to manage it so that we can use it to our advantage: too much and it can handicap us.

For instance, if I'm crossing the road and a lorry comes rushing towards me, I'll feel a surge of anxiety. This helps me to think quickly and to act fast. Without wasting precious time, I am able to run back to the pavement or to the other side of the road, whichever is quicker. If I didn't do that, I'd be in big trouble. This surge of anxiety is a helpful response to real danger – in fact, it is crucial to our survival. However, if I'm so worried about crossing the road that I can barely leave the pavement, then my anxiety is obviously unhelpful.

If I have *some* anxiety before giving a presentation, the adrenaline will help me to keep focused, think sharp and it will give me the stamina to get through. However, if my fear is so great that it stops me from thinking straight, then again my fear is unhelpful.

So you can see that anxiety and fear are helpful responses – sometimes even lifesaving – but you can have too much of a good thing. The skills you'll learn from this book will help you manage your anxiety so that it works well for you, rather than causing you problems.

Our ancestors and stress

Our ancestors evolved to deal with very tangible threats to their safety, such as a charge from a wild animal or an attack from a hostile tribe. It was lifesaving to be alert and able to respond to stress: to fight or to take flight. This mechanism has persisted, so if modern man perceives a threat, his mind and body are prepared for it by a surge of adrenaline. Even if the stress we face is not physically dangerous, we have the same response that our ancestors had.

We often feel stressed when our safety is not actually threatened – if we are late, or have domestic problems, or a deadline or an exam is coming up, or we have too many things to do in too little time. Relationship problems can also cause a great deal of stress, as can financial worries. Even things that are meant to be pleasurable and happy, such as weddings, holidays or parties, can cause such stress that these occasions no longer feel like something to look forward to, or something that will be fun. In response to those stresses, we can feel 'wound up', irritable or afraid, even though none of these things is truly dangerous – all because our bodies and minds have interpreted a threat and are preparing us to deal with it.

What happens to our bodies when we feel stressed?

Let's go back to Marie and her son. She felt nervous, shaky, began to breathe quickly and found it hard to swallow. These are just a few common sensations people feel when they are stressed or anxious. We might also feel general muscle tension and some of us find our blood pressure rises temporarily. We might break out into a cold sweat, feel flushed or feel sick. Sound familiar? Each of these reactions – even if they don't feel productive or helpful – reflects a bodily change which gets us ready for action so that we can deal with a perceived threat. Physical tensions prepare our muscles to work, while rapid breathing ensures there is enough oxygen for the job and raised blood pressure ensures that the blood can get vital oxygen to our mind and muscles quickly and efficiently.

What happens in our minds when we feel stressed?

Marie was focused. She didn't think about the 'scene' that was going on but only about the real danger and helping her son. Nothing else distracted her.

This focused thinking is typical when we're in danger. It's an ideal state of mind for anyone facing a serious challenge, say, a pilot doing an emergency landing, or a parent grabbing a toddler who is about to run into the road. This is another aspect of the stress response that can work well for us.

How does our behaviour change when we feel stressed?

Marie saved her boy from choking without really thinking about it consciously. It felt automatic. She got up quickly from her seat and helped her son by using a technique she learned a long time ago. She was persistent and kept going until it worked. She benefited from the energy, speed and focus that the stress response can give us. Another example of helpful behaviour under stress is if I'm driving and go into a skid. I 'automatically' and swiftly grasp the steering wheel and find the strength to correct it, and I don't give up until I am out of the skid. It's a vital reaction in a dangerous situation.

UNHELPFUL OR PROBLEM STRESS

If you are reading this book, you probably are experiencing problem stress or anxiety. Problems arise when we experience the stress response when we are *not* in a truly dangerous situation or when it's exaggerated. Then, our bodily and mental reactions are out of keeping with the reality of the situation and they can begin to cause us distress. They can start to spoil our quality of life and even our self-esteem.

For example, a student might be so nervous about his exams that he can't revise properly and performs badly, which leaves him feeling disappointed in himself; a man might choose not give a presentation at work, even if it means missing out on a possible promotion, because his fear of embarrassing himself is greater than the anticipation of a more favourable outcome; a mother who is afraid of being in a confined space might not be able to go on a family holiday because being in a car, train or plane seems intolerable. As you probably know well, lives can be really limited by fears and anxieties.

Interestingly, up to a point, our ability to cope with stress actually improves with stress. You can see this in Figure 1.

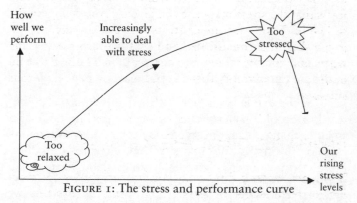

FIGURE 1: The stress and performance curve

Source: adapted from R. M. Yerkes and J. D. Dodson (1908), 'The relation of strength of stimulus to rapidity of habit-formation', *Journal of Comparative Neurology and Psychology*, 18: 459–82.

At the bottom left of the curve in Figure 1, we are relaxed but physically and mentally not so well equipped to deal with danger because we are not ready for action. As tension rises, our body and mind become primed for confronting stress. Stress and adrenaline are helpful – but you can have too much of a good thing and there comes a point when increasing stress becomes counter-productive and we are less able to cope as our stress level increases (we go over the top of the curve). Our thinking can then become too fixed, our physical responses too extreme, like the student whose mind goes blank in an exam or a person who freezes in a frightening situation. Although this is quite normal and most of us will have experienced it at some time, problems arise if we always quickly go into this state. It can become our 'default mode' and can prevent us from gaining the benefit of the stress response. Also, it can be an unpleasant and even frightening experience in itself. The key to stopping this is learning more about stress and anxiety management; that is, learning to make stress work *for* you rather than *against* you.

Stress that looks good from the outside

Look at the exhilarated faces of the people on the downwards loop of a rollercoaster or on the trading floor at a stock exchange: some people enjoy the rush of adrenaline triggered by stress and anxiety! They interpret it as 'fun' rather than 'danger'; 'harmless' rather than 'harmful'; a 'one-off' rather than a 'life-sentence'. This is not a bad thing unless a thrill-seeking person lives their life at the top of the stress curve, enjoying the thrill but always being close to becoming overstressed. Even if you enjoy stress, it's important to know how to unwind and give your mind and body time to recover – otherwise, you can be at risk of becoming too stressed and, in the longer term, stress can take a physical and mental toll on you.

Long-term stress

Sarah gave up a stimulating job to devote more time to her three young children.

> *I thought that being a stay-at-home mum was the best thing for the children, and a good thing for me, but going from dealing with rational adults*

all day to entertaining three lively, boisterous children, one of whom got up repeatedly in the night, was a shock to my system. I just didn't adjust to it very well.

The kids got up very early and then it was constant chores and breaking up rows, or dealing with tantrums, or illness. At first I had a burst of energy and I really applied myself and made sure my children were kept busy and entertained, and that I got all the housework and cooking done. But it got harder and rainy days seemed to drag on forever. What really hurt was that I was not enjoying it, as I felt I should, and I became tired, could not keep on top of things. I started to go to bed earlier, sometimes not long after the children did, because I knew I would be up with the youngest in a few hours. My immune system was shot and whatever bugs they got, I got as well, but still had to drag myself out of bed to look after them. I also had what I now see were symptoms of stress, like constant tension headaches and tummy upsets. I felt permanently exhausted and had a very short temper. I remember shouting at one of the children in a supermarket and people giving me dirty looks, and thinking to myself, 'Oh, I've become one of those mums who shout in public.' But mainly I felt tired and tearful much of the time. Permanently on edge. A good friend told me I was no fun anymore, and that maybe I wasn't cut out for this. That really hurt, and made me feel inadequate and depressed.

Sarah's experience highlights how any of us might begin to feel when we don't get a break from feeling stressed.

She was in a pretty constant state of tension which led to her having headaches and tummy upsets, feeling irritable and tired. All of this is reversible, but Sarah would have to change her lifestyle somewhat to get relief. She was also struggling because of her interpretation of what was happening – she criticized herself for not being a good enough mother and wife, and she ended up feeling inadequate and her mood suffered. The way she came to view herself actually added to her stress.

Longer term stress and the body

The bodily sensations that might be fleeting when we face short-term stress can feel more pronounced and more overwhelming if we have to endure them over a long period of time.

The **muscle tension**, so important for flight or fight, can develop into something that feels more like pain. This might take the form of tension headaches, discomfort in swallowing, shoulder, chest or neck pain, stomach cramps, trembling and weak legs. It can also lead to a sense of fatigue.

The **increased blood pressure**, which provides the brain and muscles with a much needed blood and oxygen supply, can make our heart feel like it is pounding, and we might get ringing in our ears.

The **rapid breathing** (sometimes called hyperventilation), which ensures that we have a plentiful supply of oxygen, can begin to cause feelings of light-headedness, blurred vision and nausea.

Although this physical response sounds dramatic – and it certainly can be pretty horrible if you are experiencing it – it is a natural consequence of long-term stress. When we don't engage in the 'fight or flight' behaviour, which would burn off excess oxygen and make full use of the extra muscle tension, we experience the discomforts of the stress response. Some people who feel anxious most of the time can feel unwell a lot of the time, and they might be told it is all 'psychosomatic'. It's easy to interpret this as being told that it is 'all in the mind', but 'psychosomatic' means *mind and body* – the stress might start in the mind but you will feel the effects in your body. Sometimes these symptoms of stress themselves become a new source of anxiety and a person can start to fear the feelings of fear itself.

Let's return to Sarah's story. Her energy reserves have been depleted by the effects of long-term stress and worry. She hasn't worked out how to minimize the effects of her stresses; she feels constantly worn out and less able to manage things. She's caught up in an unhelpful cycle, which is shown by the dark arrows in Figure 2: she's stressed and her stress response now undermines her ability to cope – and so she becomes more stressed. The energy which got her through the initial crisis is no longer there, and the net result is that she feels worse in her body and mind, at least for the time being. Sarah also worries about not coping and this sets up another cycle, which is shown by the thin arrow in Figure 2, and this reminds us of the role the mind plays in the unhelpful stress response.

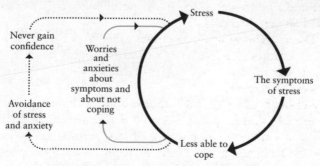

FIGURE 2: The cycles of stress and anxiety

Longer term stress and the mind

Mental changes are inextricably linked to the physical changes. If, like Sarah, you feel physically rotten, most of the time, it is going to colour your outlook and your mood – which in turn, can affect your stress levels and the way that you feel in your body.

If you are particularly sensitive to all the physical changes you feel, you might start to really focus on this and possibly misinterpret your physical feelings as something danger-ous. You might interpret a chest pain as a heart attack, a stomach ache as an ulcer, lower back pain as kidney disease or shortness of breath as lung cancer. Even if it happens time and time again, but is *never* a heart attack, an ulcer or disease, you might still think: 'Yes, but *this* time . . .' If you focus very much on your physical symptoms, it's hard to think about anything or anyone else and this keeps the cycle of anxiety going by directing your thinking towards aches, pains and odd sensations and your worries about them. This, again, is shown in Figure 2.

Some anxiety sufferers become serious worriers, always anticipating the worst – 'I'll lose my way in a new town and miss my appointment and get a reputation for letting others down'; 'Something bad will happen to the children on the school trip – I might never see them again'; 'I am going to be so overwhelmed by anxiety that I'll make a fool of myself and be the laughing stock of the meeting.' Worriers are 'What if . . . ?' thinkers. A worried travelling companion tends to be the one asking: 'What if the passports are lost? What if we miss our connection? What if the hotel wasn't booked properly?' This state of mind can become a habitual outlook that will also fuel the stress cycle.

Some people who feel anxious and worried much of the time might also become irritable, constantly fearful and ultimately demoralized. Sometimes it is much easier to see this happening to someone else than it is to see it in ourselves. If you have toothache and are snapping at everyone, someone else is going to point out your sour mood to you (if he or she dares) but all you notice is the toothache. Consider if this is happening to you and try to manage your stress before your relationships suffer and, very probably, give you more to worry about.

Longer term stress and behaviour

We're programmed to try to make ourselves feel better. When we're cold we put on a sweater; when we're hungry we eat. So, when we're stressed, we automatically do what we can to ease those feelings – even if it is not a good long-term solution. Imagine two young women sharing a flat. Both have recently been made redundant, and both are worried about paying next month's rent. One takes comfort in overeating while the other loses her appetite completely and starts living off coffee and cigarettes. Both are stressed but they behave in quite different ways from each other, each doing something to try to ease the stress. It's possible that their responses are so automatic that they are unaware that what they are doing is responding to the stress. Someone else might try to ease their discomfort by turning to drugs or alcohol, or by working too hard, or by doing superstitious things like following a strict ritual or carrying a lucky charm in order to feel more confident.

Although these things seem to work in the short term, their use can actually prolong or add to the initial problem by threatening our physical well-being or our relationships. Clearly, one tub of ice cream is not going to harm you, but if you comfort eat that much every night, it's not going to do your body (or your self-esteem) any good. Most importantly, though, not only do these distracting and/or comforting ways of behaving cause further problems but they also prevent us from addressing the real trouble. In the short term, this understandable *avoidance* of facing the problem can give some relief but if it's not addressed, it can sometimes get worse. This is shown as the broken line in Figure 2.

Avoidance

One of the most common behaviours in the face of stress is avoidance, that is, physically leaving or never going into a situation that causes stress or anxiety. We probably all know someone (it might be you) who rarely ventures out of the house to social events, or walks many flights of stairs rather than get into a lift, or drives only on minor roads, avoiding motorways. In a situation that causes anxiety, it often seems easiest to avoid or leave the situation. So the 'nervous traveller' decides not to travel at all, or the person who feels anxious in closed rooms stands by the door or just walks out.

Jack was anxious and couldn't enter classrooms. He quickly learnt the attraction of avoidance: 'If I stand by the door I still feel very sick and nervous, but if I actually walk out of the classroom, within minutes I feel better.' The thinking which drives avoidance goes like this: 'If I stay in this situation, I'll continue to feel bad. If I leave, I will feel better. So I'll leave.' The possibility of staying and feeling better, at that moment, is inconceivable. However, leaving or avoidance do not work in the long term. In fact, they make fears worse because they stop us from learning that we can cope and this reinforces anxiety. It is the 'crash dieting' of anxiety. It works for a very short while, but it does not address the real fear. As Jack discovered:

> *The trouble is, I can't walk back in without feeling bad again. I know it's only a matter of a metre or so, and I ask myself why I feel bad on this side of the door, but OK on that side of the door. I don't know why. I do know if it carries on I will have to leave school.*

If you look at Figure 2 (p. 17) again, you can see all the links between feelings, thoughts and behaviour in the stress cycle, and how they all feed into one another. When anyone gets locked in these patterns too easily, a normal anxiety response can turn into problem anxiety. The cycles can be broken, but it does take work, dedication and self-compassion. Understanding how these cycles apply to you will be important to your success in overcoming your difficulties and so we will be returning to them again in the next chapter.

2

UNDERSTANDING MORE ABOUT PROBLEM ANXIETY

We have seen that problem anxiety can arise when a person gets caught up in vicious cycles of fear, stress and worry. It also happens when a person is simply oversensitive to threat so that the slightest suggestion of a threat (even if it's actually not that likely) can be enough to trigger anxiety. In addition, it can become a problem if the anxiety response is exaggerated and disproportionate to reality. It is at these times that the anxiety response starts to work *against* us rather than *for* us.

Reza had just this rapid and exaggerated response.

> *I just hate social gatherings – I'm afraid that I won't fit in and others will think I'm boring and a bit of a waste of space. If anyone asks me what I'm doing at the weekend, I panic even though there's no real threat at that point – but I'm really scared that I'll be invited to something social. If I do go to a social gathering, even another guest's smile will*

trigger sweating and strong feelings of anxiety because I always assume that they are laughing at me – even though this seems crazy when I get home and think about it. It's all so difficult that I tend to cope by avoiding as many social situations as possible.

This meant that Reza got caught up in the avoidance trap and he was not able to develop the social confidence he needed.

Sometimes the anxiety seems 'to come out of nowhere' but there is usually a trigger – it's just that the stress response becomes so fast and the triggers are so subtle that it *seems* to come out of nowhere.

The trigger can be a tangible threat or one we hold in mind – something we anticipate or a memory of a bad experience, for example.

Mo once felt really unwell on a particularly bumpy plane ride and then anticipated feeling unwell on his next plane journey. In fact, just *thinking* about feeling unwell on the plane made him start to feel anxious and sick even before he boarded it.

Sophia, a young woman with a phobia of lifts shied away from watching films and TV programmes that might contain scenes of a lift because the *mere image* triggered anxiety.

WHAT KEEPS PROBLEM ANXIETY GOING?

This is where we revisit the vicious cycles, which were introduced in the previous chapter. By now you'll appreciate that our thoughts have an impact on our feelings, which then affect our behaviour, which in turn affects the way we feel and the way we think – and so on. As the key to managing fears and worries is breaking unhelpful cycles, we now need to look at them in more depth: the bodily sensations, the thinking patterns, the behaviour and the circumstances which can fuel problem anxiety. When you understand the cycles that maintain your problem you'll be able to start planning how to break them.

How bodily sensations keep anxiety going

When our body tenses up from stress or fear we feel it physically, and this can fuel problem anxiety in several ways. See how many of the following sound familiar to you:

- Over time the physical sensations are unpleasant to the point of being distressing in themselves. If this has been your experience, then you might have grown to fear fear itself. Once this fear is established, just the anticipation of the physical symptoms of fear can bring them on.
- Physical reactions, such as tense muscles, shaking and dizziness, interfere with our ability to do what we need to do. So we might find it difficult to speak clearly, carry something without spilling it or sign our name clearly, for example. The realization that we can't perform as well as we want to can feed our anxieties. Anticipating that we will not perform well can set in motion the unhelpful physical reactions.
- Sensations can be misinterpreted as threatening – a racing heart can be mistaken for a heart attack or light-headedness can lead to the fear that you are about to faint, for example. Such misinterpretations fuel mental anxiety, which then keeps the physical symptoms of anxiety going. Even when you know

these symptoms are probably caused by stress, you can sometimes have a niggling feeling of 'What if *this* time, it's not stress, but something more serious?' or 'What if my nausea means I really will vomit?' Those niggling worries can also fuel the anxiety.

- The link between doing something and then having unpleasant bodily reactions can also feed anxiety. If every time you gave a presentation at work, you felt hot, sweaty, dizzy and sick, you'd create a memory of this which might be revived the next time you give a presentation, or anticipate giving a presentation. Studies show, for example, that cancer patients can start being sick as soon as they enter the room for chemotherapy – before actually being given treatment – because they associate the treatment with nausea and vomiting. So this automatic association brings on distressing physical feelings that can then feed anxiety.

How our thinking keeps anxiety going

In the previous section, it was clear that anticipation can keep anxiety going, but there are several other ways of thinking that maintain anxiety. The overall term for these unhelpful kinds of thinking is *biased* or distorted thinking. With anxiety and fear, the bias is usually on the negative side: if there is a chance of weighing up the outcomes of a situation as either good or bad, the anxious mind will tend to think the worst. It's not intentional but more of a habit, and one that can be broken.

Suppose it is the first day of a new job. You set the alarm early, but for some reason it doesn't go off and you wake up late. Your anxiety will be raised, and immediately you start to think about how terrible it will look if you're late on your first day. You have to get dressed in a rush and you put on a shirt that isn't ironed properly. Now you think your new colleagues are going to think you're a slob as well as late! You know if you skip breakfast, you can just about make the train that will get you to work on time, so you grab your coat and keys and rush out of the door. Anxiety can affect memory and halfway down the road, you realize you've forgotten your briefcase. You rush back home, grab your case and run out again. You can't remember if you locked the door. You're now anxious, distressed and worried about leaving the door unlocked for the day. You think about the alarm, the shirt and the briefcase, and start to blame yourself. You're now feeling highly stressed and your mind races: 'What else will go wrong today? It's all gone wrong so far, it's bound to get worse!'

While you could be forgiven for thinking that many people would react with similar levels of distress to all this, there are some people who would shrug it off and think: 'I've done my best in the circumstances', or simply, 'Things will probably get better.' Others would be mildly distressed but feel comforted that they will at least get to work on time, so the shirt and unlocked door don't matter so much, or they would say to themselves: 'I bet I'm not the only one wearing a creased shirt', or 'I've probably locked the door but I can ring Jeff and ask him to check it on his way to work.' But some people who have a *negative bias* in their thinking will continue to think 'What if . . . ?' and imagine a whole host of other disastrous things that could unfold because of their difficult morning: 'What if they judge me on the basis of my shirt?'; 'What if they think badly of me?'; 'What if I get burgled?' As a result, they're going to feel increasingly anxious. The more anxious they feel, the more biased their thinking – it becomes a vicious cycle.

WHAT TYPE OF THINKING MAINTAINS ANXIETY?

A particularly powerful mental 'engine' for driving anxiety, which you saw in the example above, is a combination of:

- *Overestimating* the threat to you.
- *Underestimating* your ability to cope.

These really feed the anxious thinking cycle. If you *overestimate* the likelihood of failing an exam and *underestimate* your intellectual ability, you're going to feel pretty nervous which might then affect your performance; or if you *overestimate* the dangers of driving on the motorway and *underestimate* your driving skills, you might avoid driving and never build up confidence in your ability to drive.

When we get distressed, we are all prone to extreme and biased thinking – but if this becomes a habit, it can become a source of anxiety. How many of these common types of anxiety provoking thinking have you experienced?

1. *Ignoring the positive* – letting achievements slip by you, missing compliments or not being able to get an optimistic perspective.

2. *All or nothing thinking* – it will be great or terrible, it's a total success or a total failure, with no in-between.

3. *Exaggerating* – related to 'all or nothing' thinking, but always leaning towards how bad things might be.

4. *Scanning* – constantly looking out for signs of the thing you fear.

5. *Catastrophizing* – seeing the worst-case scenario.

6. *Selective attention* – similar to ignoring the positive, this means having a bias towards noticing the negative, such as focusing on the only disappointing thing in an otherwise great meal that you have made.

7. *Jumping to conclusions* – mind-reading and fortune-telling.

8. *Self-reproach* – blaming and criticizing yourself.

9. *Worrying* – getting caught up in endless 'What if…'s.

Being aware of these biases is really important so we'll look at each of these more closely. Again, see if you can recognize these thought patterns in yourself – without judging yourself! Just see if you are nodding in recognition.

Ignoring the positive

This is common in depression as well as anxiety. It means that we filter out the good things that might have happened or might happen and just focus on what went wrong or what can go wrong. This can really colour our view not only of the particular situation but life in general, because this kind of thinking easily becomes a habit.

If you've generally had a good day at work, but your boss comments on a minor mistake you've made, the mistake is what you bring home with you if you ignore the positive. The rest of the day, with its good elements, is forgotten and as a result you end up feeling demoralized and your confidence takes a beating (see Figure 3 below).

To combat this kind of thinking, you need to be able to appreciate your strengths and achievements and keep them in the picture, and this book will help you to learn how to do this. It might sound odd, but it can also help to talk

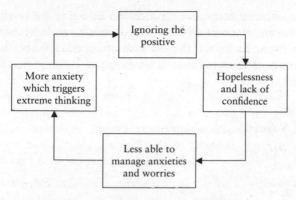

FIGURE 3: The 'ignoring the positive' trap

to yourself as you would to your best friend, or a child. If a child brought home a school report that was mostly As and Bs, with one D, would you focus on the D or on the good grades? What is going to make the child feel better if they are only looking at the D? You'd say, 'Hang on, what about all these great grades? This tells us that you've got a good brain.'

You, too, have a good brain. Never forget that your anxiety can be managed, and it is unhelpful to chide yourself for the things that you can't do right now. Focus on the good bits, so the bad bits don't start to feel so overwhelming.

All or nothing thinking

This means seeing everything as extreme, with no moderate or in-between option. It's not unusual – you see this in teenagers, when everything or everyone is either awful and terrible, or amazing and brilliant. It is a style of thinking that can be triggered in any of us when we feel there is a threat. For example, seeing a child run out in front of the car would trigger a helpful 'life-or-death' thought, which would spur us into action to save the child. It's also common in perfectionists: something's got to be done perfectly or not at all.

In those who suffer from problem anxiety, this type of thinking can become a habit and, as the thinking tends to be towards the more alarming option, it drives anxiety. Also, always thinking in the extreme gets in the way of taking a balanced viewpoint and getting on with problem-solving (see Figure 4).

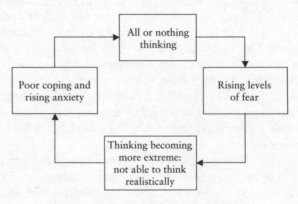

FIGURE 4: The 'all or nothing' trap

The strategies in this book are not going to encourage you to combat negative thinking styles by simply replacing them with positive ones, but will encourage you to take a more moderate view and consider more realistic possibilities, possibilities which take in a range of options, not just extreme ones.

Exaggerating

Exaggerating means magnifying the worst aspects of an event, person or situation. An anxious person might always focus on the worst things that happened and then make them seem bigger, such as: 'It was *absolutely* awful. *Everything* went wrong and *no one* knew what to do. The event was a *complete* disaster and I was *utterly* hopeless – couldn't do a thing, a *total* waste of space'; 'It was the worst flight ever. Unbelievably bumpy, hit many, many air pockets. We could have crashed'; 'This time, I really, really did think I was going to die!'

Thinking about what happened in an exaggerated way will make the situation seem a lot worse than it actually was. This just feeds right back into the cycle of anxiety (see Figure 5).

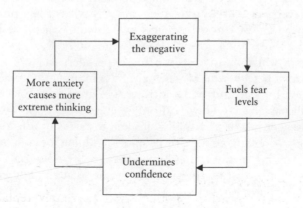

FIGURE 5: The 'exaggerating' trap

It's important to be aware of the language you use because words which exaggerate, such as 'completely awful', 'absolutely hopeless' and 'totally terrified', can lead to exaggerated thoughts.

It's also possible to exaggerate in anticipation of an event and predict a worst-case scenario: 'I *will* fluff my lines'; 'The diagnosis *will* be cancer'; 'My son *will* injure himself badly'; or 'The house *will* catch fire.'

Scanning

When countries are on a health alert, because of a flu epidemic, for example, it's interesting to see how people react: most of us start to scan for signs of danger. We really pay attention when a friend says that they aren't feeling well, and we notice if someone takes out a handkerchief – are they going to sneeze? We focus on possible threats. And it affects our behaviour: when someone sneezes, we give them a very wide berth, more so than usual. Some people even put scarves over their mouths when using public transport. We can all engage in scanning when we feel under threat – it's normal. Usually the public fear subsides after a while, and we stop being hyper-alert. However, an anxious person who worries about contamination will be driven by fear and will continue to scan a train for signs of ill passengers. They will only feel reassured once every passenger has been visually checked for signs of infectious illness – looking sweaty, or pale, or trembling, or coughing.

Scanning means being hyper-alert to any noise or smell or sound or feeling that might indicate 'danger'. Someone with a spider phobia will visually check all the corners of the room and anywhere else that could harbour a spider. A person with a phobia of thunder will scan the weather reports and will be on the lookout for dark clouds. Someone with health anxiety might scan the newspapers for signs of the latest bug that is felling the workforce and start to scan his own body for symptoms: 'I've got a bit of a headache. That's one of the signs! I think I'm coming down with it!' In contrast, another person, who does not have health anxieties, might read all the news stories, get a bit of a headache, take a paracetamol and simply think: 'I've got a headache.'

A major complication of scanning is that it increases our awareness of worrying things which would otherwise have escaped notice. Being on the lookout for danger means that there is more of a chance that 'danger' will be noticed – an ache in the body, a spider hiding in the corner, a look of contempt on the boss's face. This increases the likelihood of feeling anxious – no trigger is unseen – and it fuels the fear, as you can see in Figure 6. Even worse, in a heightened state of fear and worry, misinterpretation is common and so we can get alarmed by harmless things. For example, a normal ache will be interpreted as a sign of a serious health problem; a harmless shadow on the wall can be mistaken for an intruder; a stifled yawn might be seen as a look of contempt. If you really look for something, there is a good chance that you'll find it, even if it's not actually there.

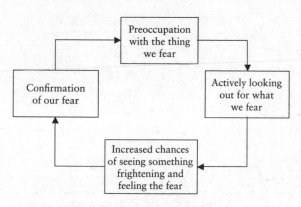

FIGURE 6: The 'scanning' trap

Catastrophizing

This simply means anticipating disaster as the only possible outcome. Like all the other thinking biases, it's often difficult to spot this when you are doing it because it's so automatic.

Fancy trying that new restaurant? 'No thanks, it's always empty so the food's probably really dodgy. They might not pay much attention to the preparation and be unhygienic – I could catch a bug and then I won't be able to finish my project at work and then my boss will criticize me . . .'

Do you want to go out tonight? 'No, the weather forecasts rain and it'll be impossible to get a taxi home, so we'd be stuck in the bad weather we've been having, and then I'll be late getting home and then I'll probably oversleep in the morning . . .'

And it's possible to catastrophize for others: 'You're going for a minor operation? I've just read an article about someone having a rare allergic reaction to anaesthetic and going into a coma, so it's not just MRSA that you need to worry about . . .'

A very common form of catastrophic thinking is about physical symptoms or minor ailments. So a lingering headache, to the catastrophic mind, is almost certainly the first sign of a brain tumour. A lump is sure to be cancer. A sore arm is first sign of a heart attack.

Catastrophizers tend to get caught up in the cycle shown in Figure 7.

This can really limit your options and you will do fewer things, because you predict possible (imagined) disaster. Doing fewer things means that you won't be building your self-confidence that you can cope: another vicious cycle which maintains fear and anxieties.

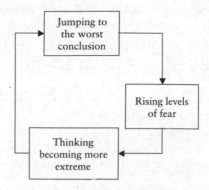

FIGURE 7: The 'catastrophizing' trap

Selective attention

When we pay more attention to a particular aspect of a situation, we are showing selective attention. For example, if you buy a new Ford Mondeo, the chances are that you will selectively notice other Mondeos until the novelty wears off. That's not harmful – just human nature. So, as with so many of the things we've talked about, it's a normal reaction. However, it becomes unhelpful if selective attention persistently draws our attention to what we fear.

Philip was scared of heights: 'Whenever I plan a car journey I think only about the bridges which we'd have to cross and I become anxious just contemplating the trip – I lose sight of the pleasurable aspects of a journey.'

Rhonda had health anxiety and she paid selective attention to, and remembered, the day's aches and pains rather than what had been effortless and painless.

Richie was over-concerned with safety and feared doing something which might lead to his home being damaged:

I'm in a constant state of 'red-alert' at home. If I sit down to watch TV, my attention drifts almost immediately and I notice shadows on the walls and worry that this might indicate rot. I find that I'm studying electrical appliances to check that they've been switched off at the main socket and I notice 'hot' smells which might suggest an electrical fault – in short, I've created a lovely home which I'm not able to enjoy.

In Figure 8 below, you can see how this can feed into a cycle of selective attention and fear: how this way of thinking can maintain anxiety by always directing attention to what we fear.

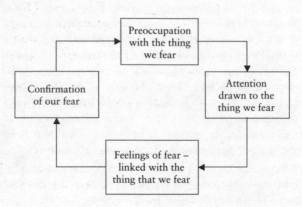

FIGURE 8: The 'selective attention' trap

Jumping to conclusions

The problem with jumping to conclusions is that we are influenced by 'gut feelings'. Sometimes these are helpful but if we are afraid, our 'gut feelings' can tell us that some-thing is more threatening than it really is: 'I *just know* that there will be an accident'; 'It's going to go terribly wrong – I *just feel* it'; 'She thinks I'm stupid and not up to the job: *I can tell*.' The two main types of jumping to conclusions which can give us grief are: *fortune-telling*, when we make a prediction based on nothing but a feel-ing; and, *mind-reading*, when we presume what someone is thinking.

Vera was preparing for an interview:

> *I was made redundant nearly a year ago. At first that was a relief, and I chose to take some time just recovering from the stress of it all. Then I dis-covered that there are not many jobs around for a woman of my age and with my qualifications and I'm very aware that an employer will see that I haven't worked in months. At the interview tomor-row, they are bound to think no one has wanted to give me a job, that I'm a dead loss [mind-reading] and I just know that they won't be interested in me [fortune-telling].*

In this case, Vera did get the job and concluded, 'They must have been hard up for applicants and thought they'd bet-ter take me rather than leave the job open [mind–reading]. I expect that they'll want to replace me as soon as they can [fortune-telling].' Here we see that Vera fell into the trap of jumping to negative conclusions (see Figure 9) both before the interview and even afterwards when she had the job. This sort of thinking will keep her fear levels high and, in turn, this will cause her to predict the worst – even though she has no hard evidence, just her 'instinct'.

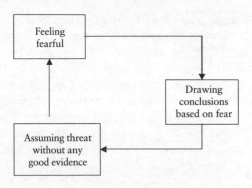

FIGURE 9: The 'jumping to conclusions' trap

Self-reproach

This happens when we let the 'inner critic' or 'bully' take centre stage. When we tick ourselves off ('You've only got yourself to blame!'; 'You should have done better!') and call ourselves names ('Idiot!'; 'Weakling!') we just make ourselves feel less confident and pessimistic. Criticism does not help anyone overcome fears, which is why self-compassion and kindness are stressed so much in this book. The 'self-reproach' trap is shown in Figure 10. The most effective way of breaking this cycle is by being accepting, non-judgemental and constructive towards yourself. Then, when things don't go well, you will stand a better chance of being able to review what happened, learn from your experiences and plan how to do things differently next time.

Worry

We are all familiar with this term and a certain amount of worry can be helpful if it directs our attention towards a problem that we can solve. For example, if you're worried

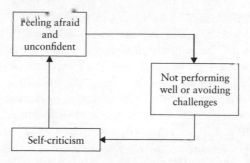

FIGURE 10: The 'self-reproach' trap

about forgetting a passport before a trip, this might prompt you to write down a checklist of things to remember; if you're worried about your car breaking down, this might prompt you to book in an overdue service; if you're worried about missing a deadline, this might give you the impetus to work particularly hard and to meet that deadline. Problem solved.

However, if worrying does not lead to constructive problem-solving, but just to a series of 'Oh dear . . . what if . . . ?' questions then it will fuel anxiety.

Cassie had a twinge in her tooth. Her partner suggested she visit the dentist. 'But what if he finds something wrong?' Her partner suggested that the dentist would fix it. 'But what if I have to lose the tooth?' Her partner suggested that this was unlikely and even if she did she could have a replacement. 'But what if it's really expensive?' Her partner reassured her that they could afford it. 'But what if I got an infection?' You can imagine how the conversation progressed. With each 'What if . . . ?' she became more anxious and more prone to worry – and her partner became more frustrated.

A series of 'What if . . . ?' questions does not lend itself to problem-solving. None of us can problem-solve a question – we need to name the fear. In Cassie's case this might be: 'He could find something wrong and then I might have to have some serious, and potentially expensive, dental work.' This gives us something to work on and we stand a chance of addressing it. Unfortunately the person who is prone to worry tends not to clarify the fear but moves on to the next 'What if . . . ?' and their anxiety escalates.

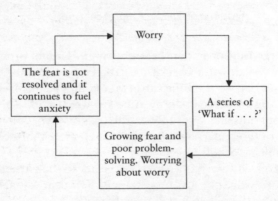

FIGURE 11: The 'worry' trap

Sometimes people worry out of habit and sometimes it is to avoid naming the bigger fear. Cassie was actually avoiding stating that she was afraid of having a bad reaction to dental anaesthetic and ending up with brain damage (an example of catastrophic thinking going hand-in-hand with worry). The stress of her comparatively minor worries was easier to bear than contemplating her worst fear. However, if she doesn't name her real fear she cannot address it.

Sometimes people worry because they think that it's a useful thing to do: 'If I worry then bad things won't take me by surprise.' But this still results in a pattern of thinking that will maintain an anxious state of mind.

Whatever drives the worry, the worrier gets caught in the worry trap (see Figure 11). Sometimes the worrying becomes a worry: 'All this worry will drive me mad/harm my health'.

Thinking biases often occur together. Peter had low self-confidence and assumed that others would find him boring or stupid. In work and social situations, he would *scan* people's faces, looking for signs of disapproval or boredom. His *selective attention* meant that he didn't notice smiles and nods of approval, and his tendency towards negative *exaggeration* meant that the slightest sign of disapproval was magnified – his *all or nothing* thinking then transformed this into an extremely upsetting experience: 'He really thinks that I'm stupid and worthless'. Thus, Peter often misinterpreted a harmless expression as a judgemental one and then his thinking became *catastrophic*. He predicted that word would get round that he was stupid and then people would be less likely to want to know him and his boss would question his capability . . . and so on. Afterwards he would be beset by *worries* about the incident: 'What if my boss does think I'm not up to the job . . . ?'

It's easy to see how powerful a thinking style can be in maintaining worries, fears and anxieties. However, the coping strategies in this book can help you manage this.

WHAT KIND OF BEHAVIOUR KEEPS ANXIETY GOING?

If you have read other books on anxiety, fear or worry, you might have come across the term 'safety behaviour' to describe a response that maintains anxieties and fears. Safety behaviours start out as a way of making us feel safe but, in the longer term, they stop us from learning the skill of coping. They include having a drink of alcohol for 'Dutch courage', carrying a lucky charm, or maybe carrying out a comforting ritual.

There are two safety behaviours, in particular, which can be really effective in fuelling fears and anxieties: avoidance and seeking reassurance. It's natural to try to avoid what we think is dangerous or to look for reassurance about our worries and this is fine – *up to a point*. If you experience anxiety on underground trains, you can avoid that anxiety by avoiding underground trains – but if that stops you from learning to manage your fear, then it's a problem. If you're worried about your health and turn to your spouse for words of comfort, you might feel relieved in the short term, but if this reassurance prevents you from learning to calm yourself, then it's a problem.

Avoidance and escape

There is an old joke in which a man says, 'Doctor, doctor, I can't do this,' as he tries to lift his arm. The doctor shrugs and says, 'So don't do it.' This can be one of the assumptions behind avoidance: that the problem can be dealt with by ignoring it. But the most common assumption is that it is just not possible to cope with the stress or distress of facing a challenge: 'I'll never mange to do that without going to pieces'; 'I couldn't possibly take that on – I'd freeze up and look a fool'; or 'If I tried I'd only fail and feel even worse.'

As you know, avoidance does not resolve problems: fears are never overcome and avoidance itself can cause more problems. However, it's a popular coping strategy because it gives short-term relief – that's why so many people keep turning to it but it is a poor coping strategy for the longer term.

As we saw in the last chapter, avoiding something reinforces the idea that *not* doing something is a good strategy for dealing with anxious feelings. For example, everyone knows that Jane from accounts doesn't 'do' lifts. She takes the stairs. But when she has to go to a meeting in an office on the twenty-sixth floor of another building, she might find that not 'doing' lifts presents her with a major problem.

Some avoidance behaviours are small and thus acceptable as 'quirks' at first, as in Jane's case, but the more you avoid something, the harder it becomes to face that challenge and the more complicated things can become.

Jonas never travelled far from home because he feared using public transport and being away from home. Over time he became less and less confident about travelling. This might have been OK (although boring) for him if he'd lived alone and his job didn't require him to travel: but he had a family who wanted to go on holidays and his boss wanted him to work away from home from time to time. His avoidance of travelling prevented him from developing the confidence he needed to face these challenges and the prospect of tackling them became worse and worse. This created additional stresses – domestic tensions because his wife and children were unhappy that they never took holidays together, and work-related problems because his boss was becoming irritated by Jonas's lack of commitment to his job.

Avoidance wears many disguises

Avoidance is not always easy to spot: it can be well disguised and subtle. It can be passed off as something else. So the person who is afraid of going to the cinema might say, 'Oh, there's nothing I want to see,' or 'I've heard that film is rubbish.' The person who feels anxious going to the shopping centre might say, 'I don't really enjoy shopping. It's handier to do it online.' It can seem more socially acceptable than admitting that anxiety is the problem but these sorts of excuses lead to the types of behaviour that maintain the cycles of anxiety and fear.

Avoidance might appear in more subtle forms. Perhaps the person who feels ill at ease in the cinema will still go but only if he can sit by the door for a hasty exit, or after he's had a drink to 'calm his nerves', or if he's carrying a lucky charm, or if he's followed some sort of reassuring ritual like getting dressed in a certain way before going out. Maybe the person who fears the shopping centre will still go shopping but only with a good friend, or only if she can use a shopping trolley to steady her if she feels that she might faint, or only at extremely quiet times. In each of these instances, the anxious person in not learning that they can actually manage the task – so their fears remain unchallenged.

Sometimes, a socially acceptable stimulant, such as tea, coffee or chocolate, will be used to 'get through' a stressful time, as they are often distracting in the short term. We often offer these things to people who look like they need a break, or are worried or upset. Although they are largely harmless stimulants, and ones which most of us enjoy, they do trigger the release of adrenaline, which is *not* good for someone who is already anxious. Other people will turn to alcohol for 'Dutch courage' and it might work in the short term, but later on it actually makes the stress worse by disrupting sleep, causing dehydration and, if overdone, resulting in a hangover. The other problem with using these substances to get through is that you never really find out if you can manage without them. But you can and this book will show you ways of combating avoidance.

Seeking reassurance

We all want to be soothed and told that there is a way through this problem – it's an instinct from infancy. We particularly want to be assured by people we know or love, or whose expertise we trust, such as a doctor. There is nothing wrong in turning to others for support and advice that will help us learn to deal with our difficulties – the problem with reassurance (repeatedly seeking assurance) is that it doesn't work in the long term because it actually stops us from learning how to assure ourselves. Some people describe it like a 'fix' – a few reassuring words from a partner or a professional and everything feels OK – but, like a 'fix', the feeling does not last. If reassurance really did work, people wouldn't feel the need to come back again and again with questions like: 'Do I really look OK?'; 'Tell me again – will everything be fine?'; 'I did lock all the doors, didn't I?'; or 'Could you just look at this again, doctor?' People who repeatedly seek reassurance are not really taking on board the assurances, so deep down they remain scared and therefore they look for comfort again. This can be quite frustrating for the people who have to do the reassuring and it can put a strain on relationships. When this happens, there is the danger that worrying about the quality of the relationship will then add to stresses and insecurity.

The Internet, offering the possibility of looking up symptoms at a glance, has created a new monster which is sometimes called 'Cyberchondria'. If you're prone to seeking reassurance, it can be tempting to seek it 'online'. An initial gathering of information to use to help assure yourself is fine, but returning to the computer to get that 'fix' will only make things worse in the longer term. In addition, there is a lot of misleading and inaccurate information on

the Internet and you could end up even more worried than
ever.

THE THINGS AROUND US THAT KEEP
ANXIETY GOING

So far, this section has focused on the feelings, thoughts
and behaviours which keep anxiety going, but we all know
that sometimes external stresses and the actions of others
play their part, too. There are things going on around us
that can add to or help to maintain the anxious thought
cycle. These tend to boil down to:

- *Circumstances* like stressful periods at work, long-
  term unemployment, financial pressures and illness.

- *Interpersonal stresses* such as domestic problems and
  relationship difficulties. These might well put anyone,
  not just anxious people, under extra stress.

It's not always possible to avoid these things, but once
you learn how to think and behave in a way that doesn't
fuel anxious feelings, you can cope better with these life
events.

She means well, but . . .

There is one particular interpersonal situation that can
cause difficulties for an anxious person, but which is hard
to recognize because it involves kindness and helpfulness
on the part of the other person. For example, a mum who
is developing agoraphobia might ask a neighbour to do the
school run for her. The neighbour understands, and brings

this woman's children to school – which seems helpful but it allows the mother to avoid her fear and prevents her from overcoming her agoraphobia. The man who's terrified of giving a presentation at work asks his colleague to do it for him – if the colleague agrees, then this man does not tackle his performance anxieties. A student who's terrified of driving on motorways might get his girlfriend to drive him around but, comfortable as he feels, he's not overcoming his fear.

These 'helpful', well-meant responses are actually keeping anxiety alive because the anxious person does not learn to assure themselves and develop the confidence that they can cope. In all these situations, it's better for the friend or family member of an anxious person to offer emotional support and encouragement, but not to take on the task of their anxious friend. A really helpful response would be, 'I understand you have difficulty taking the children to school. Would it help if we walked together at first?' The colleague who has agreed to take on the presentation might say, 'I realize this is a problem for you, and I will be happy to help you prepare and you can rehearse with me, but I think it's best that you give it a go yourself.' The girlfriend who has agreed to chauffeur the student around might say, 'I know it's a scary thing. I was afraid of motorways as well when I first passed my test, but the more you do it, the easier it gets. I'll come with you.'

You can still be honest with your friends and family about your levels of fear – it's important that they appreciate that you are truly scared and not being lazy, for example – and accept their support, but make sure that *you* are dealing with your worries, rather than allowing other people to help you avoid them: this will be the most effective way of overcoming your fears.

BREAKING THE CYCLES

The great thing about identifying the cycles which keep problems going is that you can start to see where you can break them. Now you have read this chapter, take a moment to review what you've learnt about the vicious cycles which you get caught up in:

- What physical sensations might keep *your* fears and worries alive?
- What thinking styles or thought patterns resonate with *your* own way of thinking?
- What behaviours might be making *your* problems worse?
- How might circumstances or other people be playing a part in maintaining *your* anxiety?

When you have identified the patterns which maintain your anxiety, you can start to think about breaking these unhelpful cycles in the ways described in later chapters in this book.

The next chapter considers who is at risk of anxiety-related problems and why. This will help you to understand why you might have developed your difficulties, and this might help you to be more compassionate towards yourself if you tend to be harsh. Being less harsh on yourself can be one way of breaking unhelpful cycles.

3

WHY SOME PEOPLE ARE MORE PRONE TO ANXIETY THAN OTHERS

It isn't essential, but it can be useful to understand where your anxiety, worries and fears might have come from. Of course, this insight won't solve the problem but it can help you appreciate that there are reasons that you have your difficulties and that it's not just your lot in life or just your fault.

Jane says she comes from a long line of worriers:

My mother worried about everything, and her mother did as well. She had a hysterical way of talking, and if my brother or I got a cut or scrape or fell over, she would get very nervous and whip out the first-aid kit and talk about infection and all these things that scared me. She used to dwell on terrible stories of things that happened to children in the neighbourhood. This one got run over by a car, that one's appendix burst and he nearly died. It was often her main topic of conversation.

My grandmother's favourite book was a home medical encyclopedia. She was always looking for signs and symptoms of illness in herself and her family, and also came out with these stories about Mrs So-and-so down the road who was in the queue at the bank and just dropped dead from a heart defect nobody knew about.

They both seemed obsessed with other people's illnesses and I was determined not to be that way myself. But when I had my own children, any sign of a snuffle or bad tummy and I was straight off to the doctor's. I constantly think something bad is going to happen to the children. If the phone rings at work during the day and they say it is a personal call, I always imagine that it is the school ringing to say there has been an accident involving one of my children. I am constantly on edge. I'm sure it's affecting my performance at work. Sometimes I start to shake and I just tell people I've had too much coffee. I wish I could be one of those people who are just relaxed and calm.

NATURE OR NURTURE?

If Jane was telling you this story over coffee, you might well say, 'I blame the parents,' and in some ways you might be right. Jane says her mother and grandmother were obsessed with catastrophe and seemed driven to focus on tales of woe. Her brother, Josh, grew up in the same environment, but he is not a worrier. He jokes that worrying is the family curse, but that it is in the female genes, as he takes after his more laid-back father. It is interesting that two people who grew up in the same environment were affected so differently. This might lead you to conclude that it is nature (in the genes), and not nurture (influenced by a person's environment and the way they were brought up), that predisposes someone to anxiety. However, it might have been the exposure to all those stories of medical horror which resulted in Jane's fears – stories which Josh didn't listen to. We just can't know.

An anxious person is not necessarily 'hard-wired' for fears and worries and it's too simple to 'blame the parents'. There are many ways a person might develop an anxiety disorder, and most psychologists think that a combination of factors cause this: nature, nurture and specific life circumstances.

As we saw earlier, understanding the development of our fears can stop us from simply blaming ourselves or simply blaming others, neither of which is productive. What *is* productive is taking a non-judgemental stance and considering why it's *understandable* that we have certain difficulties, and then using this understanding as a basis for developing coping plans.

In looking more closely at the source of your worries you might identify patterns of behaviour and thinking from the past that still cause you problems in the present, even though your situation has changed. For example, a little girl who went to a heavy-handed dentist and experienced considerable pain might continue to experience fearful thoughts about the dentist and she might still avoid going well into adulthood. Her situation might be completely different now, but the fearful feelings and the urge to avoid going to the dentist can remain the same. Realizing this can help her appreciate both why it's understandable that she suffers from dental phobia and why she's not conquering it: 'It's no wonder I have this fear – my times at the dentist were really scary and any child would have been afraid. I still have predictions about how awful the dentist will be and so I often cancel my appointments – no wonder I'm not getting over my fears yet: this is what I need to tackle.'

Having said this, sometimes it is not possible to explain the development of anxiety problems with confidence and we have to accept that we might never fully understand 'Why me?' This is not a huge obstacle as coping is very much based on understanding what *maintains* the problem now rather than what *caused* it.

Whatever hand nature or nurture or life circumstances have dealt you, it's important to remember it's an explanation, not a 'life sentence' nor a 'get-out clause'. It might be tougher for you to cope if, like Jane, both nature and nurture seemed stacked against you, but that does not mean you can't overcome anxiety. By all means, consider what might have helped to cause your anxiety, and certainly note what kind of behaviour might be keeping it going, but, most crucially, remember that many sufferers find that they have the power to get over it.

WHAT'S AT THE ROOT OF YOUR ANXIETY?

There are several risk factors for developing problem anxieties, fears and worries. The most common are listed below. The more of these you 'tick' the more you can say it's understandable that you've had some difficulties:

Family history: does anxiety and worry run in your family?

Life stresses: are you having to deal with a lot of pressures and demands – even happy ones such a promotion and marriage?

Personality type and general outlook: some people just

seem to be less laid-back than others, while others are more pessimistic (the glass is 'half-empty'), less philosophical (less likely to say, 'What will be will be, don't fret over it') and more likely to be stressed or fearful. Chapter 9 will help you be realistic in your outlook.

Coping strategies: using unhelpful coping strategies or not having enough good ones will increase the likelihood of having anxiety problems. Fortunately, this book will help you develop a wide range of good techniques.

Support network: the less social support we have the more likely we are to have emotional difficulties. Social support can help to protect against such problems and so it's really important that you ensure that you make the most of your support network – therefore the next section will look at this in more depth.

Support network: we all need somebody

Who are your friends? Who can you turn to if you need help? This is an important question as close relationships with friends and/or family can help reduce emotional problems. If you have someone to confide in, someone you feel close to, you'll be less vulnerable if you have anxiety-related problems. Though good support networks and great friends are an extremely valuable asset to anyone going through a hard time, it doesn't mean that the more friends you have, the less likely you are to experience anxiety in the first place – the benefit of a support network comes when you *use* it. One reliable friend who you can talk to is better than a large network of people in whom you cannot confide. So when you have difficulties, you should consider talking about them. Get some of the issues worrying you off your chest, and maybe get another point of view.

But don't lean too heavily

That said, it's important to get a balance in your relationships. Don't lean so heavily on friends and family that you over-invest in the help of others and then fail to develop the skills and confidence to cope by yourself. And be sensitive to the other person's resources – they may not always have the time or the emotional energy to offer support. This doesn't mean that they don't care, but they can't always be available. This is another good reason for not relying too heavily on one person – instead, try to build up a support *network* of several people. It is, of course, very important to check that you are not falling into the trap of seeking reassurance from your friends and family or using social and domestic activities as avoidance strategies.

Still, having good friendships and developing a support network will help you cope with many of the problems life throws at you – and it's also just a really nice thing to do! It makes life more enjoyable. However, a tendency with anxiety, like depression, is to cut yourself off from friendships or any social situation that might provoke distress. Instead, be open with your friends about your problem and don't pull away from friendships because of it.

4

WHAT KIND OF ANXIETY PROBLEM DO I HAVE?

Anxiety disorders come in many forms, but some have such a distinct pattern that they have their own labels. While it can be helpful to have a label for what you're struggling with, naming it does not mean that you're saddled with it: you *can* break free of it.

The most common anxiety problems are:

- Simple phobia
- Agoraphobia
- Panic disorder or attacks
- Health anxiety
- Social phobia
- Generalized anxiety disorder
- Obsessive compulsive disorder
- Post-traumatic stress disorder
- Burnout

Although some of these terms might be familiar to you, some might be new to you so we'll look at each of these in turn – if you see your own difficulty, or aspects of your difficulties, in the descriptions then this can help you better understand your problem and that's the beginning of seeing your way through it.

SIMPLE PHOBIA

A phobia, sometimes called a 'simple phobia', is an intense fear which is out of proportion. Phobias might be focused on things that most people regard as unpleasant (vomiting, for example) or potentially dangerous or painful (like bees, which could sting) – but most people view these concerns as a part of life, not something to be avoided at all costs. Some phobias are rare, such as button phobia, but for the person with this phobia the feelings are always intense and often disabling.

The labels for specific phobias can sound very exotic as they are generally named after the thing that is feared, using the Greek vocabulary. For example:

apiphobia: fear of bees   *arachnophobia*: fear of spiders
brontophobia: fear of thunder   *emetophobia*: fear of vomiting
haematophobia: fear of blood   *hydrophobia*: fear of water
ophidiophobia: fear of snakes   *ornithophobia*: fear of birds
zoophobia: fear of animals

Such is the intensity of some phobias that the sufferer not only avoids the thing itself, such as wasps, but even pictures of wasps or even the word 'wasp' – as pictures and words can sometimes trigger the fears. Fear could also be triggered by sounds, for example, the humming of a refrigerator might remind someone of wasps sufficiently to set off a powerful anxiety response. A person with a phobia tends to use scanning as a means of coping – and as we've already seen this can make things worse.

Pippa recalled:

> *I know exactly how my phobia started. I was five, in school, and was suddenly sick, and all the children laughed or made signs like they were disgusted and filed out of the classroom holding their noses. The teacher told me off. Since then, I've been afraid not only of being sick myself, especially in public, but of other people being sick in case it makes me sick. The noise, the smell, the feeling that it will never stop, the lack of control – all these things completely terrify me. I've since learned through websites that this is a common phobia but quite difficult to overcome completely, possibly because nobody actually likes being sick and it's really unpleasant for anyone. Learning that I'll be OK even if I vomit would improve the quality of my life as I do avoid many situations where I might come across someone who's being sick, such as closing time at the pub, or airplanes, or hospitals. I'm always on the lookout for people who look like they might be sick. I hate leaving the house when the 'winter vomiting virus' is doing the rounds and I restrict my eating so that if I do get it, I won't be very sick, and I try not to go into work. I avoid foods like rice and chicken and eggs in restaurants, because I've heard these have all caused outbreaks of food poisoning in the past. Now I'm also worried that my husband is getting fed up and resenting having to deal with the children every time they are sick. I'm also really afraid I'll pass on my phobia to them.*

Pippa vividly remembered the distress of being humiliated and upset at school. This was the beginning of her extreme fear and she has built her life around minimizing the risk of vomiting, developing many 'safety behaviours' which are actually making matters worse. She has now developed a collection of new worries: that she might risk her job if she takes too many days off work for fear of catching bugs; that her relationship with her husband is strained; that her children might follow her example and 'learn' this fearful behaviour.

AGORAPHOBIA

Contrary to popular belief, agoraphobia should not be defined as just a fear of leaving the house. The term describes a fear of an anticipated threat in a situation where there may be no easy means of escape. Very common predicted threats include having a panic attack whilst away from home (panic attacks are described in the next section), or collapsing in the street, or becoming confused and lost. These predictions are often catastrophic – the person thinks that the worst possible outcome will happen. Sometimes the sufferer cannot quite pinpoint what the danger is, but they have such a strong sense that 'something bad will happen' (jumping to conclusions) that they try not to leave their place of safety 'just in case'. As avoidance leads to loss of confidence, someone with agoraphobia will get worse by staying where they feel it's safe.

Michael was always a very sociable person. He worked in the music business, a job which involved lots of travel and lots of late nights:

In my job, I often had to go on the road with bands. I was the one who stayed sober and responsible, to make sure the band got to places on time. A while back I was working with one particularly difficult client: she was very moody, very rude and everything I did was wrong. I was already exhausted and needed a break and I started to get very anxious around her and I had several panic attacks at particularly stressful times when I had to be really together, like checking in for a flight, or checking in to a hotel, or taking her to a television appearance. She really humiliated me and I felt worse than ever. This tour was the longest three weeks of my life. I lost weight and felt constantly ill. I thought I actually was ill, but when I got home my doctor told me it was a form of 'nervous exhaustion'.

I took a month off. I felt so much better not being under pressure. Then a record company called me and asked me to take on another tour. Just getting ready to go to a meeting about this made me start to feel panicky. I realized I hadn't really gone anywhere for a while and didn't know if I could cope. I made myself go but I had to leave the meeting room twice because I was gasping for breath. I was embarrassed and I thought: 'There's no way I can travel with a band if I can barely function at this meeting!' Afterwards, I was shaky and exhausted and I went home and went to bed. I've turned down every job which involved travelling since then and I only take work which I can do from my office. I'm worried that I will have a panic attack in public so I do a lot of my food shopping online.

Despite my taking it easier, I have actually grown less confident about going out. I don't feel *that I'm the person that I used to be and the thought of being in some situations makes me anxious and shaky. What I fear most is having panic attacks again. My doctor says I have agoraphobia. I'd always thought agoraphobia was something stay-at-home-housewives got, not people in the music business.*

For Michael, one bad patch at work had very big consequences for his mental health. He was already tired and needed a break and the additional strain of the difficult client and her humiliation of him triggered a series of panic attacks. He then developed a fear of having panic attacks. He tried his best to ease his distress by taking it easy and avoiding the challenge of travelling, but this has sapped his confidence. His thinking is now negative and he predicts that he can't cope, which erodes his confidence even more.

PANIC DISORDER OR ATTACKS

Michael was afraid of having panic attacks, which is understandable as they can be extraordinarily unpleasant, even terrifying. Typically, they involve sudden increases in anxiety along with symptoms such as:

- racing heart
- breathlessness
- dizziness

These are exaggerated anxiety or stress symptoms but the onset can be so sudden and powerful that they take people by surprise and are quite shocking. It isn't unusual to find this terrifying and sometimes the experience is made worse because the symptoms are misinterpreted as signs of a really serious physical problem such as a heart attack or a stroke, or a person may think of themselves as 'going mad': this is catastrophic thinking in action.

We say that someone suffers from 'panic disorder' if they get recurrent panic attacks. This commonly occurs with agoraphobia (as Michael's experience shows) but it can occur without it. People who have panic attacks often describe them as 'coming out of the blue' – they feel fine one moment and awful the next. However, there is usually an alarming thought that precedes the scary sensations. It's not always easy to catch or recognize or challenge that thought, and it quickly causes anxiety and a panic attack.

A common physical feature of a panic attack is over-breathing, or hyperventilation, which simply means breathing very quickly. As a result of this, a lot of oxygen enters the bloodstream and this in itself triggers sensations that can be disturbing, such as tingling under the skin, dizziness and ringing in the ears. Some people describe feeling 'unreal' or 'not quite with it', which can be especially upsetting as this can be interpreted as somehow going 'mad'.

All this sounds very alarming – and it is for anyone having a panic attack – so it's no wonder that people, like Michael, are afraid of them and organize their lives to reduce the chances of having them.

Louise, a computer programmer, had a panic attack on a recent work trip. It had a knock-on effect.

> *I was on a work trip to Manchester and though I tend to be a bit anxious, I thought I would be so busy there that I wouldn't have time to worry and I'd be able to just focus on my work. I kept myself going by having lots of coffee. I started to feel unwell and my heart was racing, and I*

*figured it was the coffee, but there was a nagging
doubt – was it a heart attack? I was in a taxi going
to the train station and I really began to feel hot
and sick and I couldn't breathe properly. The
station was very crowded and I fought my way
to the toilets. I was so scared because I really
thought that I was having a heart attack. I told
someone this and they rang for an ambulance.
At the hospital the staff eventually realized that I
was having a panic attack and one of the doctors
gave me a tranquillizer to help me calm down. It
worked enough to get me on the train home but I
felt awful and so embarrassed. I thought that it
was a 'one-off' but I began getting panic attacks
on the way to work, and at work, and just at random. Even though I know what they are, I still find
them so awful and embarrassing that I'm scared of
having them. My big fear, however, is not being
able to work. I have not been on another work trip
because my doctor will not give me tranquillizers
and I can't see myself coping without some.*

Louise can see how her panic attacks started: she had a tendency towards worrying, she was under stress, she drank
too much coffee, she became frightened by her racing heart
and her fears triggered a panic attack. She is now so scared
of having panic attacks that her anxiety is raised, which
makes her more prone to having the panic attacks – she
has developed panic disorder. She jumps to the conclusion
that she will have another attack in a similar situation, and
makes excuses so she doesn't have to go on work trips.
Unfortunately, this sort of anticipation plays a big part in
making her even more nervous and vulnerable. Her way
of coping now is through avoidance and this just saps her

confidence further. It is clear that Louise is caught up in very vicious maintaining cycles.

HEALTH ANXIETY

Some people are constantly troubled by concerns that they have, or might develop, some illness or another – perhaps this describes your anxieties. This over-concern with health matters is called health anxiety or hypochondriasis and, like other anxieties, it can result in a time-consuming and distressing preoccupation.

Health anxiety sufferers tend to deal with their worries in three ways:

- Trying to avoid thinking about health issues by not reading or talking about certain health problems.
- Looking for signs of illness by scrutinizing their bodies – searching for moles, lumps under the skin and so on (scanning).
- Reassurance seeking – asking others (doctors, family or friends) their opinion in the hope that this will put their fears to rest.

Although understandable, each of these ways of coping can actually maintain the problem; avoidance stops a person from ever learning how to tolerate the fears and distress; looking for signs of illness usually results in finding something to worry about – in fact, sometimes irritated, discoloured or raised patches of skin are caused by constant prodding and poking; reassurance usually gives only temporary relief – the nagging worries soon kick in again because sufferers come to rely on others and don't learn to assure and calm themselves.

Sophia's childhood had been stressful. She was one of four children. Her mother was prone to angry outbursts and there was constant rowing in the family. Her father tended to 'escape' to the family allotment and he spent long hours at work so the children saw little of him and his absence made Sophia's mother more angry. Sophia lived 'on edge', waiting for the next angry outburst: she never felt safe and always had a sense of 'I'm-not-really-safe-something-bad-will-happen'.

When I was ten a girl at school died of cancer. I didn't really know her but I was devastated as this seemed to prove that terrible things could happen and therefore I was not safe. From that moment on I began checking my body for signs of illness – trying to catch disease early. In my late teens I frequently begged my father to take me to the doctor. He'd do anything for a quiet life so he'd take me for regular consultations. There was never anything wrong and I'd be reassured for a while – which felt blissful – then the nagging worries would return: 'What if the doctor misunderstood what I was saying and he was wrong when he told me that I had no need to worry? I forgot to mention that I also have incredible fatigue – perhaps I do have leukaemia after all.' Then I'd want to go back and I began asking the doctors for blood tests. When I left home to live with my boyfriend I soon got into the habit of asking him to look at my skin and I badgered him with questions about illness. He was helpful at first but eventually he said that this wasn't doing any good and he's stopped reassuring me. I think I've annoyed him, so now I feel worse than ever.

As you can see, Sophia grew up in a tense environment and she developed a sense of foreboding that turned into health anxiety when the schoolgirl died. Her scanning and checking, her father's support in reassurance seeking and the 'blissful' relief she got after hearing that she was healthy ensured that the problem didn't go away. Fortunately, her boyfriend is no longer giving her reassurance – but the stress in the relationship is probably making her anxieties worse.

SOCIAL PHOBIA

Social phobia is rather different from the 'simple' phobias described (though no phobia is simple for the person who has it). People with social phobia fear situations where they might be evaluated or scrutinized by others. They typically anticipate being judged and found wanting, and find this extremely hard to bear. These social anxieties cause them to become socially phobic because they predict being distressed and not being able to tolerate it. They do lots of mind-reading and tend to assume the worst.

Anticipation plays a major part in social phobia: fear that something bad might happen triggers symptoms of anxiety that can actually make matters worse. For example, shaking, sweating, needing to go to the lavatory or not being able to think straight can all worsen anyone's performance and this can increase social anxiety.

A hallmark of social phobia is extreme self-consciousness, so there is always an element of 'performance anxiety' and mind-reading: 'What are others thinking of my conversation? I bet they think I'm boring'; 'What are they thinking about my presentation? I hope they don't ask questions which catch me out.' Sufferers are excessively aware of themselves in social settings – it's often hard for them to think beyond their personal discomfort or difficulties and so it's difficult to focus on a task or to engage properly with others or to get distracted from their social fears. This, of course, often makes the problem worse.

John has a job which involves a lot of public speaking. Though he enjoys other aspects of his job, he finds the public-speaking part very difficult:

> *Believe it or not I am the union rep for my firm, so I often have to speak publicly and sometimes to the press. It never gets any easier. I'm good at writing and good on the phone so that's why the role appealed to me, and I just thought the public-speaking part would work itself out. If I have to talk to a group I feel very self-conscious, sometimes to the point where I almost feel unreal or very detached which I have to say scares me. I also tend to feel hot and dizzy and, at its worst, my anxieties make me feel sick and I get palpitations. This distracts me and I can't think straight. All that goes through my mind is: 'I'm making a mess of this. I must be coming across really badly; everyone can see I'm rubbish.' I am acutely aware that my mind and body don't seem to work properly for me at these times. I must look an absolute idiot and others must see this. People tell me that the anxiety will ease off once I'm in the swing of the presentation – but I've never found this to be so and my fear of public speaking is becoming worse. I'll do anything to avoid a press conference and usually delegate it to someone else under the guise of giving them an opportunity. If I absolutely have to do one, I have a stiff drink and some extra*

*strong mints to cover the smell. I know this is not
a good way of handling it, but it's the only way I
have right now. My fear is that I won't get away
with this much longer.*

You might think it rather odd that someone with a fear
of public speaking would take on a role that invariably
involves it, but it's possible John didn't realize the extent of
his fear until he had to give press conferences. He has done
his best to work around his phobia but he has resorted to
avoidance (delegating presentations to others or drinking)
but, as you can see, this is not helping and he continues to
struggle. He's caught in the typical avoidance cycle, which
keeps anxieties going. He is also caught up in the cycle of
his anxieties undermining his performance, which makes
him more anxious. His awareness that his fears could affect
his career makes him worry even more.

Saroya has always said that she is 'no good at parties'.
She is a nurse with a lot of responsibilities, and her husband runs his own small business and is obliged to socialize
in order to develop business contacts. Saroya is expected to
join him, but she freezes up and worries about social events
weeks in advance:

*People at work would describe me as a cheerful
sort of person. At work I feel in control, I know
how to make my patients feel at ease, I commu-
nicate well with medical staff and I know that I
am good in a crisis. But when I have to go to a
function with my husband, I become a frightened
little mouse. The people he works with have a very
different lifestyle from me, and I can't imagine
what kind of conversations I can have with them.
When I'm with them, I struggle to think of things*

*to say and this really embarrasses me. I worry
that they're looking at me and thinking that I'm
socially inept and stupid and this makes it even
harder for me to think of what to say. In these sorts
of situations it's as if their words are echoing in
my head and I have no thoughts of my own. If
I can think, my only thoughts are: 'I don't know
what to say – they must think I'm a fool.' I am
sure that I do actually look socially inept and stupid. Sometimes I even stutter and shake. When my
husband tells me something is coming up, I start
to worry well in advance. The thought of walking
into a room where everyone is chatting and drinking and seems to know each other just terrifies me.
If I am introduced to someone, my mouth goes
dry and I can't think of anything to say. I don't
drink for fear of getting too 'relaxed' and making
a fool of myself and I try to 'escape' by staying too
long in the cloakroom or by offering to help with
practical things such as finding someone to adjust
the heating or to provide more nibbles. This means
that I can get away for a few minutes.*

*It's now got to the point where I will often pre-
tend I have a bad headache or I've picked up some
bug at work, just to get out of it. My husband
knows this and I think that he is tired of making
excuses for me. He tells me that he understands
and he makes light of it by joining in the joke that
he keeps his wife locked away from everyone. I've
never enjoyed myself at one of these dos and I
can't imagine that I ever will.*

What's interesting about social phobia is that people who
have it are often very good in other areas of life such as

work or home. Saroya feels like she has a different personality at work, she feels in control and she feels confident. In social situations she feels self-conscious and not at all in control. It's good that her husband is not critical of her fears, as this could so easily make her problems worse, but his making excuses for her means that she can avoid social challenges and her social confidence gets even lower – so he is not helping her in the long term. And her own solution of coping through avoidance further saps her confidence.

GENERALIZED ANXIETY DISORDER

Generalized anxiety disorder (GAD) is the term used to describe excessive anxiety or worry about several things, which carries on for over six months. The feelings of anxiety seem to intrude on many aspects of life and the result can be feeling 'on edge' a lot of the time. It can be very draining and it can really interfere with getting on with life. If you suffer from GAD, you will probably worry about the same things that everyone does – work performance, family and social issues, finances, health – but you will worry more and your worry will be triggered by more minor issues. GAD is particularly undermining as it tends to trigger catastrophic thinking (commonly characterized by: 'What if . . . ?' questions) and this gets in the way of problem-solving and dealing with challenges.

Sharon's children have left home. This has left her with more time on her hands, and, she feels, more time to worry:

When I try to explain to my friends exactly what it is I'm worried about, it's really everything. I tend to think of the worst thing that can happen in almost any situation and I seem to feel worried all the time. It's as if anything can set me off think-ing: 'What if . . . ?' People say this is just negative thinking but it really affects me physically, too. My muscles are always sore from being tense, and being in a constant state of anxiety is very tiring. I also don't sleep well so I always feel tired and irritable.

I can't remember how this started. I think I was a 'worrier' as a child, always frightened of anything new, and it just got worse. I fidget a lot and people say this is nervous energy and I need to learn how to relax, but I honestly don't know what that feels like. I thought I would relax and feel less worried when my children left home but I seem to fill the time with more worrying. I feel physically unwell quite a lot – that worries me, too: I worry what all this anxiety is doing to my health. My doctor says it is 'psychosomatic' but it feels very real to me. He said I should take up a hobby and learn to unwind, but I don't think that will help. I'd probably end up worrying about the hobby – 'Am I doing this right? Am I wasting my time?' To make matters worse, I am worried about not worrying, too! I know that this might sound crazy but if I worry at least I feel that I've prepared myself for the worst.

I work three days a week in a launderette and I try to make sure I'm busy, but because my con-stant anxiety makes me so tired, I sometimes can't concentrate properly. I make mistakes and I get annoyed with the customers. I know I have to do something about it, but I can't think what.

Sharon feels hopeless, and she feels confused that in this time of less stress at home, she feels more stressed than ever. She is now worried about being worried – which is a common feature of GAD – and yet she is afraid of letting go of her worrying – which is also a very common feature. Sharon is in a no-win situation and, if you suffer from GAD, you probably feel that way, too.

OBSESSIVE COMPULSIVE DISORDER

Anyone who suffers from obsessive compulsive disorder (OCD) will have fearful thoughts that drive the urge to do or think certain things in order to feel 'safe'. However, they don't feel comfortable with these responses, but rather view them as extreme or unusual.

For example, Jose feared being contaminated by germs, so he washed his hands over and over until they were red and chaffed. Although part of his mind knew that he was clean enough, he felt compelled to keep washing in order to feel absolutely free of germs – to feel 'safe'. Maeve feared that she might have an electrical fire and thus checked over and over again that all the light switches were off and all the plugs were unplugged. If she set off to go anywhere, she felt compelled to return to the house several times even though she knew she had already checked.

There are certain checking behaviours that are sensible. For example, if you are leaving your house, it makes sense to check that the gas fire or the cooker is switched off. Problems arise when the concerned thought isn't just a passing thing you act upon swiftly, but a doubt which drives a compulsion. 'I've been back into the house three times – but am I *totally* sure I turned the cooker off? Perhaps I better go back again and check.'

The most common fears are about:

- *Contamination* of oneself or others.
- *Missing something* potentially dangerous, which could result in an accident or major crisis.
- *Inappropriate behaviour*, which would be embarrassing.
- *Not being organized*, with things arranged in the 'right' way, in case this brings bad luck.

These fears drive *neutralizing* responses such as Jose's washing and Maeve's checking. These 'neutralizing' behaviours are intended to reassure and calm. What distinguishes them from 'regular' coping strategies is that they are usually excessive and the OCD sufferer typically feels absolutely compelled to do these things, no matter how outrageous or odd they might seem. For example, Robin always touched wood three times before he left a room because he was afraid that something bad would happen if he didn't.

Some people use 'neutralizing thoughts' or 'magical thinking' in response to anxiety. Whenever Jonas saw, heard or thought the word 'cancer' he became overwhelmed by a concern that cancer would strike him or a loved one. In order to feel safe, he mentally recited comforting words such as 'safe', 'healthy' and 'protected'. Other OCD sufferers might recite phrases or numbers or keep thinking of 'positive' images in order to combat the fear.

As with other anxiety disorders, there's a chain of events that keep OCD going. Once anxiety is triggered it is followed by a 'neutralizing' response and this prevents the sufferer from learning that things will be OK. By now, you will not be surprised to learn that OCD is maintained by avoidance. In this case it is the avoidance of the distress caused by worry: each time Jose, Maeve, Robin or Jonas give in to their compulsion, they are not challenging it and they never learn that washing or checking once is enough or that things will be OK even if they don't touch wood or that thinking about cancer won't cause it.

There are three common themes driving OCD:

- *A sense of responsibility* ('If something bad happens, it's my fault').
- *An overestimation of threat* ('If I have germs on my hand I will contaminate others').
- *An intolerance of uncertainty* ('I can't stand this feeling that something bad could happen – I'll carry out my ritual to make myself feel better').

These three types of thoughts drive the urges to 'neutralize' and 'neutralizing' responses keep OCD going. Kate knew this all too well:

> *My mates tease me about how clean and tidy I am, and how everything has to be in its proper place. If things aren't just right I feel really uncomfortable and I simply can't stand it. People ask me what would be so bad about having a less than perfect home and I honestly can't say – I just know that I have a bad feeling when everything is not just so. I do know what worries me about having a less than clean house – I am afraid that I will catch something which would make me ill. Then I worry that I might spread illness and be responsible for harming others. I have a routine for cleaning the kitchen and bathroom which is quite long but I feel it is necessary. I usually spend 5–8 hours on this at the weekend and 'top-up' cleaning during*

the week. It does take a toll on my social life but I just wouldn't feel OK if I wasn't confident that it was clean. I try to keep myself free from contamination by avoiding communal toilets, not sitting down on public transport, carrying anti-bacterial wipes to use if I think that public places are not clean and by wearing gloves – I wash them and my hands the moment I get home. I also shower when I get home and – this is a bit extreme – I find that I have to do this in a certain way. I have a particular ritual, and if I don't get it just right I have to start all over again. Sometimes I can spend so long getting it right that I run out of hot water and have to shower in the cold. I recently found a website which shows you how to wash your hands thoroughly. It takes quite some time to do it properly, if you do the nails as well, but I still do it three times to make sure that I am clean. I often do things three times – cleaning the loo, checking that food packets are not ripped, even plumping the cushions – it makes me feel more confident that I'm safe. I do get teased and that bothers me – but I can't stop being so careful as it feels as though so much is at stake.

Kate's story illustrates how compelling OCD behaviours can be and how they can be driven by just a 'sense' that something has to be a certain way – there isn't always a readily identifiable thought. Kate's story also reminds us how frightened the person with OCD is and that, odd as some of the behaviours might be, they are no joke. Teasing OCD sufferers about their behaviours only make things worse by adding shame and embarrassment to the mix.

POST-TRAUMATIC STRESS DISORDER

Post-traumatic stress disorder (PTSD) is a very specific stress reaction that follows a traumatic event such as an assault, a road traffic accident, a fire or witnessing a major disaster. It is quite normal to experience some distress following such things and most of us would be more emotional, perhaps more jumpy, for a while and we might avoid revisiting the place where the event took place. It wouldn't be unusual for us to find that we had quite vivid memories of the trauma and we might suffer from nightmares for a while. However, things usually settle down after a few weeks – PTSD is only diagnosed if they don't. The symptoms usually occur quite soon after the traumatic event although the reaction can be delayed.

A diagnosis of PTSD is quite rare as the sufferer has to experience certain difficulties including vivid images of the trauma which don't go away, have an increased tendency to get startled or jumpy, and avoid places which remind them of the trauma (for a source of more information on PTSD, see the 'Useful Books and Resources' section at the back of the book). Although not everyone who has suffered a trauma will be diagnosed with PTSD, some people can suffer some of the symptoms and can certainly find themselves distressed long after the trauma is over.

Vincent's car tyre blew out and sent him into a skid on a quiet country road one afternoon:

> *It happened so suddenly I didn't realize what was going on at first – I skidded then it went dark (that must have been when the car turned over) and I could hear metal scraping along the road and I could see fire (that must have been from the friction). I ended up in a deep ditch. The passenger*

side of the car was completely crushed in and I thought: 'Thank goodness I wasn't in that seat.' I couldn't get my door open because the car was squeezed so tightly in the ditch and my movements were restricted by all the crushed-in metal around me. I couldn't move my legs and I had my first panicky thought: 'Am I paralysed?' Then I noticed that water from the ditch was coming into the car – it was cold and filthy. I knew that I wouldn't drown but it was winter and it was getting dark and I thought: 'I could die here: it's a quiet road, it's dark and no one will find me – I'll die of hypothermia. This is it.' I lay, cold and wet, unable to move for an hour at least. The cold and the shock made me sort of drift in and out of awareness and I kept thinking: 'I'm dying – and it's my own fault.' Someone walking their dog found me and called for help – I was cut out of the car and spent a couple of days in hospital. Physically I was quite fit – I wasn't paralysed – but mentally I was a mess. It's been three months and I still have nightmares of being trapped in a dark, cold place. I have not been driving again. When I am with her, I ask my girlfriend not to drive down the road where the accident happened. I went there once and all these vivid memories came back – they're called flashbacks and having them is like being there all over again. When I have them, again I believe I'm about to die. It is unbelievably frightening when the memories return. They also come back when I hear the sound of metal scraping against something hard so I avoid railways and building sites as the noises there have triggered them recently. My girlfriend is worried as she says I'm not the same person – I'm so jumpy and nervous, and I am much more withdrawn and I don't want to talk about how I'm feeling about the accident in case it triggers flashbacks.

Like many who have been traumatized Vincent avoids anything that might trigger memories of the trauma. However, the more he avoids the more he loses his confidence in his ability to tolerate his memories and the less likely it is that the disturbing memories will be resolved. Although it can be very distressing, *facing* the memories of trauma whilst learning to calm yourself seems to be one of the most effective ways of dealing with them. However, if you actually have PTSD it is often best to do this with the guidance of a professional.

BURNOUT

This is a condition that occurs when someone is overloaded with stress and can no longer cope. It was first used to describe emotional exhaustion experienced by health-care workers, but it's now recognized as more widespread. Sometimes it is called 'executive stress' as it has been linked with the pressures of high-powered jobs – but this is misleading as any of us can suffer from it. Typically, someone with 'burn-out' will be very tired both physically and mentally, more emotional and quick to lose their temper or burst into tears; sometimes they will lack emotion and seem to be 'flat' and apathetic. The stresses that can contribute to burnout include: the pressure of meeting deadlines, overworking, trying to reach really difficult targets, job boredom, too many constraints, frustration and taking on too much because you can't say 'no'.

Sometimes, stress creates a buzz and a sense of excitement, and its disadvantages are overlooked. Think of the live television presenter who says he loves the 'adrenaline rush' of his work. Drive and ambition can override awareness of stress. Diana is stressed, but explains it is the culture of her workplace to ignore stress and not complain:

> *People just have to keep going. I worked in television, mainly coordinating outside news broadcasts, and we had to work very quickly and deliver stories as they were breaking, so the pressure was constant. It was really not the done thing to take time off, even if you were ill. I was getting a lot of colds and feeling generally unwell, but had to keep going for fear of losing my job, or thinking that people would think I was not pulling my weight. Outside I was keeping it together but I would get home from work, very late at night, and not have the energy to do anything but start worrying about what was going to happen the next day. I always had the TV or radio on to see what the big stories were, and I could not switch off. Eventually I got pneumonia and the doctor said that I'd become so run down that my body couldn't fight off illness.*

Burnout can creep up on you, as it did with Diana. She found her work stimulating and while it was admirable to be so dedicated to it, she came to realize that she had no 'down time', no time to recharge her batteries, and her personal life suffered. It took a health scare to make her reassess the effects of working so hard and lacking balance in her life.

OTHER WAYS ANXIETY AND STRESS CAN SHOW ITSELF

In addition to the problems we have looked at so far, there are other signs of too much anxiety and stress. For example, it can make us more susceptible to *physical ailments*. This doesn't mean disease or infection, but if the mind's stressed, the body can get stressed, too. Sometimes the term 'psychosomatic' is used to describe such ailments but don't be too quick to dismiss this as simply meaning, 'It's all in your mind' – as mentioned earlier, the term actually means 'mind-body' and it's a way of acknowledging that our mental state can influence our physical well-being. Almost any part of the body can be affected and the most common response is probably muscular tension. This causes aches and pains – tension headaches, chest pains, lower back pain, stomach cramps and even sore throats. In addition, chronic stress can make some physical problems feel worse – chronic pain or irritable bowel syndrome (IBS), for example. The good news is that addressing stress and anxiety, by using the techniques in this book, can help reduce these sorts of physical discomforts.

Another common problem that is linked with anxiety is *difficulty in sleeping*. Almost everyone will have trouble getting to sleep now and then, and it's not unusual to wake repeatedly during the night or very early in the morning from time to time – especially if we are going through a stressful time. However, if this goes on, particularly if it continues when the stressful time has passed, it can pose real problems. Often, the source of the sleeplessness is not being able to 'switch off' – with the mind racing with concerns. After several nights of sleep difficulties, and feeling terrible as a result of this, it is all too easy to worry about going to sleep. This worry then makes it harder to get to sleep so a cycle of worrying and poor sleep is set up (see Figure 12 below):

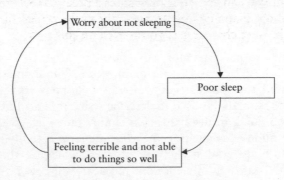

FIGURE 12: The sleep problem cycle

The driver here is worry about not sleeping and in order to break the cycle this needs to be tackled, just like any other worry (for a source of more information on insomnia, see the 'Useful Books and Resources' section at the back of this book).

WHAT TO TAKE AWAY FROM THIS CHAPTER

You will, by now, have realized that anxiety disorders take many forms and the difference between them is sometimes obvious and sometimes subtle. The advantage of working out which type of anxiety best matches your own experience is that you can often get a better understanding of what keeps it going: if you can see the maintaining cycles, you can see what patterns need to be broken.

No matter what labels we use, anxiety disorders have a lot in common, and thoughts about threat and the behaviour of avoidance, in particular, help to maintain them. Once you realize what drives your fears and anxieties, whether or not you can give your difficulties a precise label, you can set about planning how to break the cycles which fuel it.

The next chapter gets you started on this task.

5

GETTING READY TO CHANGE

As you know, the aim of this book is to help you gradually live life fully despite feeling anxieties from time to time, and for you to have a 'toolkit' of strategies you can use to feel calmer when problem anxiety does strike. It doesn't matter how long you've had anxiety problems as your toolkit will be focusing on 'here and now' challenges. It will take time and practice to get to know these methods and to work out which ones work for you best, but they should begin to take effect fairly soon into the process of learning and practising them. You will, of course, continue to experience anxiety *as this is quite normal*, but you'll have a set of strategies that will help you to cope with it and keep it in proportion.

HELPFUL AND UNHELPFUL COPING STRATEGIES

When we are anxious, we do our best to cope. Sometimes this means using strategies that get us through in the short term but which are not so good as long-term solutions – avoidance is a good example of this. A first step in managing anxiety is realizing which of your current coping strategies are helpful – you can build on these – and which you need to phase out. June's story illustrates how, sometimes, unhelpful coping strategies become a problem in themselves:

> *My mother was a housewife in the 1960s. She had a sort of vague unhappiness and nervous air and she was always going on about her 'palpitations' and 'sick headaches'. She was prescribed Valium and she became addicted. When I grew up, I was determined not to rely on medications to cope with stressful times.*
>
> *But then a series of bad things happened at once. My sister got ill and my younger son had problems at school, and I had to care for both of them. I took a lot of time off work because of this and things got tense there – they used to nickname me 'the invisible woman'. The only time I relaxed was when I got a babysitter and I could go out with my friends and have a drink. Soon, I started to drink at home as well. I thought: 'Why not? If I feel so tense and stressed and this is legal, it's not like I'm taking medication and it works, so why not?'*
>
> *I never got really drunk but I did start drinking earlier and earlier in the day, just to feel calmer. When I did not drink, I felt very anxious and unable to cope with work, appointments or any social engagements, so I'd often cancel. When I went to see my doctor about the anxiety, he asked how much I was drinking, and told me I had to cut*

down or stop all together. He suggested I read a book about CBT [Cognitive Behavioural Therapy] and, as a last resort, he offered me antidepressants which he said are meant to help with anxiety. I have mixed feelings – he's given me hope that I can manage my anxiety but I am nervous because it seems to me that this will take a long time and I'll struggle to do it without alcohol. I'll try to say no to the antidepressants as I don't want to take pills – I'm already hooked on alcohol.

June's story reminds us how attractive the 'quick fix' is, whether this is alcohol, or the tranquillizers her mother used, or the avoidance which you learnt about earlier in this book. She is understandably nervous about trying to deal with her problems without alcohol – but she recognizes that drinking is now causing more difficulties than it resolves. She is right that developing long-term solutions, such as using CBT techniques, does take more time and effort, but what she's not yet been able to appreciate is that it won't take forever and it pays off because there are no subsequent problems such as addiction and increasing loss of confidence. CBT techniques can help her to learn that she can manage her anxiety by herself. They can do the same for you.

A quick word about medication

June was offered antidepressants to help her deal with her anxieties. This is not unusual. Medications are sometimes helpful in the short term and there's no need to feel bad about taking them if you're under the guidance of a doctor. Many people find them a helpful temporary solution that can make it easier to engage with and learn the CBT strategies. If you're already taking medication and you decide that you're ready to stop, *only reduce your dose under medical advice.*

REVIEWING YOUR COPING STRATEGIES

Diary 1, at the end of this chapter, illustrates how you can collect useful information about your coping strategies and once you're aware of them, you can list them under the headings of: 'Helpful' in the long-term (I can build on these); and 'Unhelpful' in the long-term (I need to phase these out). For example:

Helpful	Unhelpful
Taking a walk, clearing my mind	Eating too much chocolate
Reading	Running away
Facing my fear	Worrying over and over
Unwinding with friends	Drinking too much with friends
Visiting the gym	Ignoring the problem
Being assertive	Criticizing myself . . . and so on

When you've done this for yourself (you will find a blank diary at the end of the book), you'll probably see that you have coping techniques which you can continue to develop and you'll spot some strategies that you'll need to phase out. It's important that you build on the helpful things that you already do as these strategies will come easily to you and probably fit your lifestyle and character. Chapter 7 onwards will give you more ideas for replacing unhelpful coping techniques, but first we need to consider what might get in the way of you being able to take to these new approaches.

TROUBLESHOOTING: USING CBT

Before you can risk changing the way you tackle your anxieties and fears, you need to appreciate just what beliefs and worries stand in the way of you making that change. Below are some beliefs which can present obstacles to recovery:

'I've never managed to get over my anxiety before. I've had counselling. I've read self-help books. I think I'm not treatable and this is just the way I am.'

No wonder you'd feel dispirited if you'd tried to manage your anxiety in the past with little or no success – but there could be several reasons to explain your lack of progress:

- *You haven't tried actual CBT approaches*: research continues to show that CBT strategies are effective in overcoming anxiety and that they're generally more effective than other psychotherapies and medications. If you've not tried CBT methods, then it is worth giving them a go.
- *You didn't give them a reasonable chance*: making changes can be testing, so try not to give up too soon. Enlist the help of family and friends who can give you support and encouragement. Be realistic and don't expect major changes at times when you're already very stressed in your life. There are many different techniques for you to try out. Some will suit you

better than others and some are more effective at certain times than at other times. Be prepared to try out a range of strategies so that you can learn what suits you and when.

- *You need the additional support of a CBT therapist*: some of you will discover that self-help is not enough and you need to be referred to a professional. This is not uncommon. If you're waiting to see a CBT therapist and want to get a 'head start', this book is a good place to begin.

'Even so, I don't know if this will work for me: is it worth the effort?'

Quite simply, you can't know until you try. A first step in beginning to get a feel for the relevance of a CBT approach is reviewing your own personal experience of anxiety – looking at your own personal pattern of it, your own triggers and maintenance cycles. There is a diary at the end of the next chapter (Diary 2) that you can use to help you do this. If you find that your anxiety is made worse by distressing physical symptoms, alarming thoughts or avoidance behaviours, then a CBT approach is worth trying.

You need to consider if the approach you choose is practical. If it doesn't fit with your lifestyle or your budget, then it won't work out for you in the long term. If you have to look after children, have no car and have limited financial resources, it wouldn't be feasible to try to manage your stress via expensive spa treatments, far from your home where there's no childcare provision. On the other hand, you might discover that your local sports centre has a crèche where you could leave your children for an hour while you swim, for a reasonable fee. It's important to plan your self-help 'programme' so that everything you try is possible with the support of others or on your own.

If the techniques in this book are going to work for you, you also need to find strategies that 'target' your particular problems. For example, if your main difficulty is coping with your physical responses to stress, controlled breathing and relaxation are good 'tools' to have in your toolkit. If you're more bothered by worrying and fears, you might find distraction techniques and learning to tackle worrying thoughts are more useful things to do. These strategies will all be explained in the second half of this book.

'But I just can't do this by myself.'

It's easy to feel pessimistic if you see yourself struggling alone. The prospect of changing your behaviours and facing your fears can be daunting but you don't necessarily have to do it alone. You might have to overcome embarrassment in confiding your fears to someone else, but do think about what you might gain from doing this. If it helps you to get started, enlist the help of a partner or a best friend or relative. Your first trips to public places or on public transport, for example, might be achieved by going with a friend. Clearly, the ultimate goal is to be able to cope on your own, but you can use help to get you there. The bottom line is that, in the end, it's better do to an activity that frightens you with a friend than to not do it at all. However, keep the ultimate goal of going it alone in mind because, as we've seen before, it is possible to become dependent on others or to strain relationships with them. Think in terms of *support*, not *dependence*.

Some readers will find that they need some professional help in order to get started or to persevere with this approach: that is not unusual and it's best to try to set this

up sooner rather than later, especially as there can be waiting lists for treatment.

'I expect my life to be changed.'

Your life can be changed by getting on top of your worries
and fears, but this book focuses on helping you to take
charge of your life rather than changing it dramatically
overnight. Expecting a speedy, major change might put
you off sticking with this self-help plan. When you think
about your goals (see Chapter 10) make sure that they are
realistic – otherwise you could get disappointed too easily
and this could stop you of making progress.

'I take medication, surely that's enough.'

Whether or not you take medication is your choice and
it's important to recognize that, for some people who are
severely restricted by anxiety, prescribed medication can be
useful, particularly if it helps them access treatment (for
example, getting to therapy appointments). It's something
you would need to discuss with your GP if you felt that
it would benefit you. It's also worth bearing in mind that
sometimes waiting lists for talking treatments (as 'therapy'
is often referred to) can be several months long, and that
medication can be helpful while you're waiting – but
reading a self-help book like this one can make the waiting
time easier, too. There is now over twenty years' worth of
good evidence that using CBT strategies to help yourself
can be as effective as using medication. It has none of the
bad side-effects *and* it has the added bonus of increasing
your self-confidence.

Diary 1

When you feel anxious or scared or stressed, note what you do and how well it works for you.

Rate your levels of distress on this scale:

0	1	2	3	4	5

Not at all scared or stressed

As scared, worried or stressed as I can imagine being

When this happened and where I was	How I felt (rating)	What I did to cope	How I felt immediately	How I felt later	What I have learnt
Tuesday: trying to leave the house without checking the locks again.	Scared 4	I went back (and then went back again) to check.	I felt such relief 1	Within half an hour I was worried again 4	It's really difficult to walk away without double- and triple-checking but it doesn't make me any less scared in the long run – it only means that I have to cope with feeling silly, too. Next time I will really try to walk away and not go back to check.

Friday morning: Waiting to go see my boss for my annual review.	Nervous 3 or 4	I kept going through what complaints he might have – thinking how I'd have to defend myself.	4	I got more and more wound up as I waited 5	Although I thought I was preparing myself for the interview, I discovered that after a point I'm just making myself more worried. Next time I'll try to distract myself when I feel that I'm just getting more wound up.
Saturday evening: getting ready to go to the party and waiting for Tom to pick me up.	Worried 3 or 4	I was tempted to cancel but I tried to stay calm and just focused on getting ready. While I waited I read my book.	2 or 3	At the party I felt OK 2 or 3	It is really hard for me to put my worries aside and to focus on something else but it pays off. It took the edge off my anxiety when I was getting ready and waiting for Tom. And later I felt pleased with myself and more confident. I didn't feel relaxed but I could cope. I will try this again.

6

STEP ONE: ANXIETY AWARENESS

IT'S ALL IN THE DETAILS: EXAMINING YOUR ANXIETY UNDER A MICROSCOPE

Of course, you are aware that you're having problems with anxiety, but as a first step in managing it, you need to look more closely to see if any patterns emerge and to discover what triggers your fear. It's a really good idea to make notes and keep diaries as experiences of anxiety can be fleeting and you may find that you quickly forget the details. It often seems as if anxiety comes from nowhere, but it's more likely that there is a subtle pattern or trigger, which you might miss if you don't keep a record. The more you understand about your anxieties and stresses, the better the position you'll be in to start to manage it.

Billy discovered more about his anxiety by keeping a diary:

> *People get afraid of certain things, but for me, it always seemed that my panic came out of nowhere.*

When I spoke with others who had panic attacks, they often said the same thing, and though it was comforting to know I was not the only one, deep down I did not really believe that this feeling came over me for no reason at all. A friend of mine was able to trace her panic attacks to a thyroid condition but my doctor assured me there was nothing physically wrong with me, which was comforting but still didn't give me an explanation. I really couldn't put my finger on what was behind my panic. It was only when I kept a diary of the panic attacks that some sort of pattern began to emerge. I discovered that they were triggered by several things, like low blood sugar, or drinking too much coffee, or when I was anxious about something else like making the right train connection I would get jittery and then I'd have the thought: 'I'm going to panic – how awful!' and that would be it: I'd panic! Once I realized better what was going on I could start to work out strategies for coping in these different situations, I felt more in control, and I could see that though the triggers were all different, they weren't random: something would raise my anxiety and that would trigger the thought that I was going to panic and then I did – it became a self-fulfilling prophecy.

You, too, can be helped by keeping a record of the times when you're feeling particularly worried, fearful or anxious. It's useful to become aware of your physical feelings, your thoughts and what you do in response to any distress. Diary 2, at the end of this chapter, shows a typical record for keeping a log of these reactions and will help you structure your record-keeping. There is a blank Diary 2 at the end of the book: there are columns for writing down where and when the fears and worries started and what the experience was like. There is a scale of '0' to '5' for rating your levels of discomfort from calm, at '0', to extremely stressed, at '5'. This is useful because it helps you to work out the different levels of your distress in different situations, particularly *after* you have tried to cope. As we saw in the previous chapter, looking back at your distress after you have tried to cope will help you figure out what helps reduce your stress, what doesn't work and what makes it worse. Remember that it can be helpful to do this twice – once immediately after you have tried to cope and again sometime later. This will help you learn more about short- and long-term coping and how effective it is for you. For example, Billy might leave stressful situations as a coping method and quickly discover that it reduces his anxiety rating in the short-term, but later, when he looks back at this strategy, he might find that his fears remain as strong as ever – avoidance hasn't really helped him. As a long-term strategy, it didn't work.

In later chapters in this book you'll be introduced to many different coping strategies that you can try out and your diary will help you get an idea which strategies work for you and which don't. Some people find it hard to rate their anxiety as it feels as though it goes from '0' to '5' with nothing in-between. With practice it becomes easier to identify the area in-between and to get a more precise understanding of your particular reactions. You just have to keep at it.

Another potentially tricky aspect of keeping an anxiety diary is that people fear that it will be uncomfortable or even depressing to see it on paper, particularly if they feel anxious a lot. Interestingly, the opposite tends to be true. Anxiety records often give you a sense of distance or detachment from the condition, and this gives you enough 'mental space' to see things differently and to start planning how to cope better.

Here are some tips to help you keep your diary:

- Use Diary 2 to get you started.
- Carry around a copy of it whenever possible so that you can catch your anxious feelings, thoughts and behaviours as they happen (before you have time to forget!).
- If you can't write things down at the time, do this as soon as you can. Perhaps you can make notes on your phone to help you remember how you felt when you fill in your diary later on.
- If you don't feel like keeping a diary, remind yourself that this is a means to an end – and that you only have to keep detailed records for a short while. Aim to keep it for at least one or two weeks.

Once you're more aware of the triggers and some of the patterns for your anxiety, you can take more control of managing it.

In Chapter 7 onwards, you'll find a set of strategies to read over, practise and then try out when you are actually experiencing anxiety. *It's important to try all the techniques, even those which don't initially appeal to you, as you won't actually know how it feels until you give it a go.* The techniques in the rest of this book tend to build on each other, so it's best to do them in the right order and to make yourself familiar with all of them.

You might have already started your anxiety and stress awareness. It will help you to get more familiar with the thoughts and feelings of fear and stress, and it should help you learn to catch your anxiety earlier, when it's easier to manage. If you've done this, it's time to move on to building up ways of dealing with the unpleasant bodily sensations and the alarming thoughts. Some of the strategies may seem familiar, and some might be ones you've already tried but which haven't quite worked. It's worth trying them again as they might be effective if you give them more time. Other techniques will be new to you, but don't be put off by the novelty, because you might find that they suit you well.

Once you've taken yourself through all of the strategies and techniques, you'll discover which methods work best for you and you will have taken the first steps in developing your own toolkit for coping. Learning to cope can be like learning a new set of skills and like playing an instrument or speaking a new language it requires regular practice. Rest assured, eventually it will become more natural and automatic and once you've got to grips with your chosen methods, you can be more confident that you can deal with the challenges that stress and anxiety pose you. You'll carry around new ways of thinking and behaving, and these are things that you'll never run out of, or lose. To make sure that you learn a 'skill for life', in the final part of the book there are strategies to keep you on the 'straight and narrow' and help you to cope in the long term.

So, as you work through the rest of this book, pace yourself and make your coping plan your own.

TROUBLESHOOTING: STUDYING YOUR ANXIETIES CLOSELY

'I know what my anxiety is about – I can skip this part.'

Maybe you're right, maybe you're very aware of the subtleties of your problem – but what if there is more to know?

By carrying out some self-monitoring you can be sure that you really understand your difficulties and then you won't risk basing your coping plans on an incomplete awareness of your problem. It's only going to require a few days of study – it's worth investing the time.

'I keep forgetting my diary and when I do remember it is embarrassing taking out a big piece of paper like that.'

It sounds as if using a copy of the diary printed in this chapter is not for you. That's fine – there are other ways of collecting information and you need to find the one which suits you. Some people find that they can speak into their mobile phone whenever the anxiety problem crops up or they keep notes on the mobile phone rather than on a piece of paper. Some people carry around tiny notebooks and use them throughout the day – then in the evening they put these brief comments into an anxiety diary which can stay at home.

'If someone saw this diary they'd think I was odd.'

You can probably keep your diary in a private place so that other people don't see it. However, to put your mind at rest you could use your own code – as long as *you* know what your messages mean it will be a useful record.

Diary 2

When you feel anxious or scared or stressed, note how you feel, what you do and how well it works for you.

Rate your levels of distress on this scale:

0	1	2	3	4	5

Not at all scared or stressed
Calm

As scared, worried or stressed
as I can imagine being

When this happened and where I was	How I felt (rating)	What was happening in my body and my mind	What I did	How I felt (rating)	What I have learnt
Monday: running late taking the kids to school.	Stressed Angry 4	My chest was tight, all my muscles tense. I kept thinking – I've got to hurry, I can't afford to be late. Everyone's getting in my way!	Ignored my daughter's advice to 'Chill out, Mum.' Just gritted my teeth.	More stressed and angry 5	My daughter's right – but I don't know how to calm myself at the time – the tension is so physical and the panicky and angry thoughts just keep rushing in. I do need to learn to 'chill out' as things just get worse if I don't. I think that I was getting stressed earlier and I just didn't notice – I'll try

Wednesday: in the shower - saw a new mole.	Panic 5	My mind raced with thoughts about cancer. What if it is cancer? What if it's untreatable? What if my kids lose their dad?	I got my wife to look at the mole. She said it was tiny - she'd noticed it before and there was nothing to worry about.	Relieved at first 1 In the afternoon, worried again	When it comes to health worries, my mind goes into overdrive if I think I've got cancer. I don't think straight at all - I jump to all the worst conclusions. My wife's really helpful - but even her good advice doesn't really put my mind at rest. I feel so embarrassed about this. I need to find a way to calm my thoughts.
Saturday: in the café waiting for Cathy to meet me. One of the customers has two dogs.	Scared 4	My heart's pounding. One of those dogs could come over here then I wouldn't be able to cope. I'd go mental. I can't deal with this. I've got to get out.	I walked out of the café and waited in the rain.	A bit shaky 3	When I see a dog I always feel afraid - I'm not even sure what I fear - I just have this bad feeling and I've got to get away. It always helps to get away but I know that, if anything, I'm getting more scared as time goes by and there are fewer places where I feel safe. I need to talk to my mum about this.

7

DEVELOPING YOUR COPING SKILLS: TAKING CHARGE OF BODILY SENSATIONS

As you now know, anxiety can cause bodily changes, which can be alarming, and someone who is prone to anxiety can also interpret normal bodily sensations as somehow dangerous – catastrophic thinking, once again. Bodily changes can also get in the way of us doing what we want to do so it's helpful to gain confidence that you can tolerate – and manage – the various physical sensations that we can all experience when we get anxious. Then you'll be less catastrophic and less limited by your physical state.

Diary-keeping: as we have discussed in previous chapters, this is always a first step in taking charge of your problems. Monitoring your physical sensations and discovering that headaches, stomach cramps and so on seem to relate to certain situations or to ease of their own accord can help you on the road to letting go of the fears that these sensations indicate something sinister. You can use Diary 2, illustrated at the end of Chapter 6, to collect information about your physical symptoms or you can design your own chart.

CONTROLLED BREATHING

This is an extremely useful, subtle and simple strategy for returning our breathing back to its normal rate and it's a technique which you can carry out pretty much anywhere, whenever you need it.

You already know that when we're anxious our breathing increases and this is normal as our body is trying to get more oxygen to our muscles just in case we need to go into 'flight or fight' mode. Sometimes this increased breathing causes changes in the way we feel physically: we can feel a bit light-headed, or get a tingling sensation under the skin, for example. Again this is normal and the sensations will pass. However, if these sensations make you feel distressed they can fuel your anxiety. One way of dealing with this is by taking steps to get our breathing back to normal as soon as we can. This is called controlled breathing. Simone used controlled breathing to help her:

> *People would point out to me that my breathing sounded 'funny' but I would never notice until I started to get really panicky, with a sore chest and tingling limbs. Sometimes I thought: 'Oh, sore chest, sore arm, heart attack!' and that made it worse. The way I eventually managed to control these sensations (which meant that I also managed my panicky thoughts) was to get my breathing back to normal. You think breathing comes naturally but I had to learn a new way to breathe when I felt anxious – but this put me back in*

control. Now I can recognize when I'm breathing too quickly and I can start to get my breathing back to normal straightaway. It saves a lot of misery and it also gives me something to focus on.

Simone describes typical 'anxious breathing' which is often called hyperventilation or over-breathing. You might assume that the extra oxygen we get from over-breathing is a good thing – and you'd be right as long as that oxygen was used up in 'fight or flight'. However, if your body doesn't use the oxygen right away, it has side effects which are not harmful but they can be unpleasant and alarming for anyone who is sensitive to the physical sensations that can result from hyperventilation.

The effects of having too much oxygen in the bloodstream can (but don't always) include:

- Tingling sensations in limbs or face.
- Dizziness.
- Difficulty in catching your breath.
- Exhaustion.
- Chest pains.
- Muscle tremors.
- Nausea.
- A feeling of being unable to swallow.

You don't have to have health anxiety to find these sensations alarming. These feelings alone can increase anxiety and cause more hyperventilation. This pattern often forms part of panic attacks, but it can happen when we are scared or stressed even if we don't have an actual panic attack.

If hyperventilation contributes to your anxiety, the good news is that it's easily controlled by breathing differently when you're stressed. Instead of breathing rapidly, you can learn to breathe *gently*, evenly, through your nose, filling your lungs completely and exhaling fully and slowly. Being more aware of how you are breathing will make it easier for you to catch hyperventilation in its early stages and, even if you don't think that hyperventilation is your main problem, gentle breathing is calming and it will certainly prevent some of the symptoms of over-breathing. For those of you who have been to a yoga class, this pattern of breathing will be familiar and you will probably have had the experience of it bringing the body and mind to a calmer state.

In order to do controlled breathing you'll need to use your lungs fully rather than your upper chest alone. When you first practise, it's a good idea to lie down so you can better observe the different way your abdomen and upper chest move. As you become more used to it, it's good to try the exercise sitting or standing, which is more likely to reflect how you will be when you'll need to use it.

1. Place one hand on your chest and one hand on your stomach. This is to help you feel the different movements of your stomach muscles and your upper chest.

2. As you breathe in through your nose, allow your stomach region to expand with air. This shows you are using your lungs fully. This is the type of breathing that is generally practised in yoga and meditation.

3. Slowly and evenly, breathe out through your nose (as your breath will be smoother and more controlled than if you use your mouth). However, do breathe through your mouth if you have a cold.

4. Repeat this in-breath and out-breath, trying to get a rhythm going. Aim to take eight to twelve in-breaths and out-breaths a minute. Don't get too caught up in trying to time it precisely but you could try practising counting five to seven seconds for each cycle of breath (breathing in

and out). Some people find it relaxing to count silently to themselves during the breath, but others just fall into the rhythm quite naturally without counting. Try it both ways and see which suits you.

Once you feel confident in taking charge of how you are breathing, you can start to use controlled breathing whenever you realize that your breathing is speeding up and you're feeling stressed. As well as minimizing unpleasant sensations, it's a soothing and distracting activity. If you use it, see how effective you have been in managing your stress and write this down in your diary. In this way you can work out how helpful the technique is for you.

It used to be suggested that you should breathe into a small paper bag to combat the effects of hyperventilation. The aim was to restore the oxygen/carbon dioxide balance by recycling air that is rich in carbon dioxide. In theory this should do the trick but it's far better to learn how to self-correct over-breathing just by slowing it down and taking smooth, even breaths. Also some people carry a paper bag around as a safety behaviour – almost like a lucky charm – and we have already discussed how unhelpful this is in the longer term. This reminds us of an important point: when you learn to take charge of your breathing pattern, remember to reflect on how *you* are developing a coping skill which *you* can choose to use under some circumstances – the breathing exercise (or the paper bag) is not managing your anxiety, *you* are. Use the breathing exercise to *build* your confidence, not undermine it.

RELAXATION

When our bodies tense we can experience pretty uncomfortable bodily sensations (various aches and pains, trembling, digestive discomfort and so on). These can be unpleasant, to say the least, and sometimes they can give rise to new concerns: 'Am I having a heart attack?'; 'Am I about to faint?'; 'Everyone can see me shake and they're thinking I look stupid!'

A good way to control muscle tension is to learn how to relax in response to it. This probably sounds obvious but it's not always as simple as it might at first appear. Relaxation is a skill and, if you're going to be able to use it when you are tense, it needs to be one that you're very good at. Below is a series of relaxation exercises for you to try out: you'll need to practise and rehearse them until you feel able to 'switch on' the relaxation response with ease. This means that you will have to dedicate time to your practice so you can't really combine it with watching TV or doing some chore or hobby. You'll need to set aside certain times every day when you do nothing but this exercise. Once you can relax during your practice periods, you can start to take on the challenge of learning to relax in response to feeling anxious. You will probably find that once you learn how to release muscle tension, your mind will follow. It's quite hard for the mind to stay tense when the body is at ease.

Preparing to relax

1. Read through the exercise instructions first as you will not be able to read and do the exercise at the same time. You can then start to work through the routines, which get progressively shorter. Sadly, there are no short cuts: you do need to practise in order to develop the skill, and the approach doesn't work better if you go through it quickly. Indeed, it can be counter-productive because you are not becoming *skilled*, you are just going through the motions. Realistically, you need to think in terms of weeks, not days.

2. Decide on a regular relaxation time that will suit you. If you work outside the home, what's the first thing you do when you get home? Increasingly, people look at emails or texts, or listen to the answerphone. Before you do *any* of that, you could do your relaxation exercises and get your evening off to a good start. You could link your practice to any routine such as brushing your teeth, getting out of bed, arriving home, for example, but do the exercise before or after one of these regular activities, not during it. Some people practise relaxation before going to sleep, but this might not be the best time to *learn* the technique as it tends to promote sleeping. In the early stages of learning how to relax, you need to associate it with getting rid of tension, not going to sleep. Having said that – if your goal is simply to go to sleep more easily, then use these exercises for that purpose.

3. Practise the routine several times a day. The more you do so, the more easily the skill will come to you when you really need it.

4. Find somewhere peaceful where you won't be disturbed. Put your phone on silent. If you have a lock for your room, use it. If you have young children (or even older ones) tell them not to disturb you for fifteen to twenty minutes unless it's urgent.

5. Make sure that you're comfortable – don't practise when you're feeling hungry or if you've just eaten, or if the room is too hot or too cold. These are distracting and potentially uncomfortable sensations that will make it harder to relax.

6. Start the exercise by lying down in a comfortable position. Later on, you will be practising while sitting or standing, which will better prepare you for the situations where you're likely to need it.

7. Don't worry about 'doing it right'. That will just add

to your worries. Just try to exercise without judgement or concerns about it being wrong or right.

8. Try to breathe slowly and evenly through your nose, filling your lungs completely so that your abdominal muscles stretch. Go back to the last section if you need a quick refresher on breathing smoothly.

9. Record your progress to see if this technique is working for you. Use a record sheet like the one at the end of the chapter to keep details of your experiences. You will have day-to-day variations. If you are less successful one day, don't be put off, but try to understand what might have made it more difficult for you that day.

The basic exercises

There are three basic exercises for you to try and they build on each other so try to work through them one at a time. The first is a lengthy exercise (although should only take ten to twenty minutes), the next is shorter and the final one is very brief.

Lengthy relaxation

This is based on a well-established relaxation routine, called Progressive Muscle Relaxation (PMR), which was developed in the 1930s and is still popular today. It aims to help you achieve a 'deep' level of relaxation using a series of 'tense-and-relax' movements that focus on the body's major muscle groups. Keep-fit fans will have some experience of tensing a muscle (say, the muscles of your bottom) in order to firm up that muscle, but that's not the aim here. The aim is simply to notice the sensation of tension, then let go in response to this.

You will work through your body from feet to head. The basic movement which you use at every stage of the exercise is as follows:

Tense your muscles, *without straining* and without holding your breath, and concentrate on the sensation of tension. You need to hold the tension for about five seconds and then let go of the tension for ten to fifteen seconds. Spend a moment or two noticing the feeling of relaxation, allowing a pleasant heaviness to enter your limbs. Imagine yourself sinking into a chair or a bed.

Feet and legs: straighten your legs, point your toes towards your face (flexing your feet). Let go, relax, let your legs go limp, and repeat.

Abdomen: tense your stomach muscles by pulling them in and up, as if steeling yourself for a punch. Let go, relax and repeat. It might be tricky to coordinate the smooth breathing with this one, but with practice you will be able to.

Shoulder/neck: shrug your shoulders, drawing them up and in. Press your head back gently. Let go, relax and repeat.

Arms: stretch out your arms and hands. Let go, relax, and let them go limp. Repeat.

Face: tense your forehead and jaw. Lower your eyebrows and clench your teeth hard. Don't worry about what it looks like. Let go, relax and repeat.

Whole body: now tense your entire body – feet, legs, abdomen, shoulders, neck, arms and face. Remember to keep breathing and hold the tension for a few seconds. Let go, relax and repeat.

It's important to repeat the exercise until your whole body feels relaxed. For some of you, this will be an entirely new sensation especially if you have spent most of your time tensed up, ready for 'flight or fight'. It can feel odd, as if you have somehow let your guard down or it can be uncomfortable to focus so much on bodily sensation. Perhaps you are already used to examining the feelings in your body, but these exercises will help you focus on feeling good, not bad.

Eddie recalls:

> *My wife booked a family holiday in America, which was a seven-hour flight. My first thought was to use a tranquillizer but I had been trying out relaxation exercises at home and wanted to try this instead. I have to admit that I'd been doing this rather half-heartedly, but then I had a real incentive to practise, so I did and it made a big difference. I discovered that relaxation was ideal because I was confined to a seat and could do the exercises unnoticed. It also felt good to tense and relax my muscles while having to sit in one seat for so long. It got my circulation going. I found it more helpful to do the long version because it took up time and, for me, it was effective. At one point we hit an air pocket and everyone on the plane gasped, but I managed to keep my anxiety at bay. That was a very proud moment for me.*

What's particularly inspiring about this story is that Eddie had tried this method, dismissed it and then returned to it because he had a real incentive to try it out. If something doesn't work the first time, it doesn't mean it will never work. Some techniques will work better than others, depending on the nature of the anxiety and the timing of a particular challenge. For this fearful flyer, an ability to relax at will was enough for him to be able to manage a long-haul flight without needing to use tranquillizers.

Shortened relaxation

Once you feel confident that you have mastered the technique of the lengthy relaxation, you can shorten the routine by missing out the tense stage. You will still need to learn to let go of tension, but without dwelling so much on the tense sensations. Go through the sequence just as systematically, relaxing the different muscle groups one by one and then, once you've got used to doing it this way, you can start to make the exercise more challenging and more appropriate for real life. For example, you could try the exercise while sitting instead of lying down, or you might move into a room that is slightly less peaceful. You can begin to learn how to relax in different places and situations – in the end this will help you cope in real life.

Bruno realized that the relaxation techniques could help him:

> *I didn't like the idea of sitting still and doing these relaxation exercises. When I feel uptight I like to ring a friend and go out – to the cinema, to dinner or to an exercise class. The idea of being still and quiet did not appeal to me – it is counter to the way I usually cope. When I really thought about it, though, I realized that keeping active as much as possible wasn't the solution for me – it wasn't working. So I gave relaxation a go. It was difficult to get into at first because the early exercises took about twenty minutes and it was very hard for me to be still and to focus on relaxing – but I accepted that I would get distracted and I refocused on the exercise. It did take some time to master, weeks, really. I am glad I stuck with it because, even though a nagging doubt kept saying that this was*

*not the right technique for me, it was – and now
I feel more in control of my tensions. I can do the
shortened version of relaxation when I need to and
it does help calm me down. Sometimes the anxiety comes back, but I just do the exercise again.
I don't expect everything to work every time, but
compared to six months ago, I feel much better
and less ruled by anxiety.*

Bruno's story shows how relaxation methods can be portable, and you don't have to rely on friends or leisure activities
(like watching a film) to help you let go of tension. Enjoyable
films, dinner with friends and exercise classes are all good
and you should think about how to incorporate more exercise and fun into your life. But you need to try to have a
combination of fun activities *as well as* the ability to relax.

Even shorter: a simple relaxation routine

This is a really brief exercise that you can practise as you become better at relaxing. It's based on an effective meditation-
inspired exercise that was developed by a cardiologist in
the 1970s. To carry out this exercise, you'll need to find
a restful word, sound or image to use during the routine
– this is common in some forms of meditation. Take your
time in finding the right relaxing image or sound *for you*.
Popular choices include the word 'calm', the sound of the
sea or an image of a favourite painting, ornament or soothing scene. It is a very personal thing and you might have to
try a few words or images before you know the one that
works for you. If you're really struggling to come up with
something, ask a friend or partner to help you come up
with ideas – but remember that it has to work for you and
not just for them! Once you have found what does work

for you, start practising by sitting in a comfortable position with your eyes closed. Imagine your body growing heavier and more relaxed, then:

1. Breathe through your nose and become aware of your breathing as you breathe in. As you breathe out, think about your relaxing sound or image. Breathe easily and naturally.

2. Let other images just come and go and simply return to your soothing sound or picture. It's natural to have other thoughts come to mind – don't worry about it, just return your mind to the exercise. This isn't meditation (though there are some aspects which are similar to it) and there is no need to try to empty your mind of other thoughts.

3. Stay with this exercise until you feel relaxed. This might take a few minutes and the time taken will depend on how practised you are and how tense you were to begin with. When you do finish, sit quietly with your eyes closed for a few moments, and then with your eyes open. Don't stand up or begin moving around too quickly – make the most of feeling relaxed.

This is a shorter exercise than the previous ones so you can practise it more often. You can do it during your meal breaks or on your way to work (but not when you're driving!) or tie it in with something you do frequently, for example, if you have regular tea breaks, then maybe do it before, or instead of, having the tea.

Lynne was worried about going to interviews:

> *There was a pattern to my anxiety. It would start to build up days before an interview, and I wouldn't sleep well and I'd lose my appetite. On the actual day, I'd feel so physically sick and tense*

that I just wanted it to be over. I think this really affected my performance and I was worried that I was not getting jobs because of my nervousness. I realized I had to work out a way to relax, and do it not only in the interview but in the days before it. To give myself a reasonable chance to learn the techniques, I asked my neighbour to take the children during my evening practice when they were home from school – this made a big difference.

At first, it was quite difficult to think of a scene other than those of previous interviews, but I told myself that this was understandable and I tried to think of something soothing. Eventually, I thought of something my mother had said to me after I'd done badly on a school exam. She said, in a very calming voice, 'Never mind, there will be more chances and next time can be better.' I'm sure lots of mothers say this but mine would give me a cuddle and really focus on me. I remember it made me feel calm and safe and hopeful. So my soothing image was of my mother cuddling me, and if I could conjure up my mother's voice, it worked even better. I learned to relax myself by sitting calmly, breathing smoothly and thinking of my mother's reassuring cuddle. I began to enjoy the exercises as it gave me times in the day where I took some time out to feel good.

When I had been practising for about a month, I was called up for a job interview. In the days leading up to the interview I used my image and calmed my breathing each time I felt tense and as a result I slept and ate better. I felt more relaxed and, moments before I went in, I just did my exercise again and the tension and sick feeling left me.

I didn't get the job, but it wasn't because of my nerves this time. Now I feel more confident that the more interviews I go to, the easier it will get.

Lynne's image was very personal to her. It was a soothing image from her childhood that brought back memories of her mother's face, her voice and her touch – no wonder it worked so well. The most effective images tend to be those which are linked to a sense of being soothed and which include sight and sound and touch. Remember, you might have to try a few scenarios before you hit upon the one that works for you.

Relaxation on cue

Now you have learnt the three main relaxation exercises, it's time to think about how you can put relaxation into action just when you need it. The first step is experimenting to see if you can do it on demand. To begin with, your cue to relax doesn't have to be a feeling of anxiety – it just needs to be a prompt to remind you to relax. Prompts can be things like getting into your car, standing in the queue for the check-out, looking at your watch, waiting for the kettle to boil or standing at a bus stop. They should be something you do or see fairly regularly and then this will step up the number of times you practise brief relaxation and will prompt you to relax at a variety of times and in different situations.

When you're aware of your cue, simply:

1. Drop your shoulders.
2. Check your breathing.
3. Un-tense the muscles in your body.
4. Bring your soothing image to mind.
5. Relax.

TROUBLESHOOTING: TAKING CHARGE OF PHYSICAL SENSATIONS

'This isn't as easy as I thought: I forget to practise.'

Bear in mind that you're trying something new, perhaps even challenging the habits of a lifetime, so it isn't strange that you forget to use your diaries or to practise your new breathing and relaxation exercises. However, if you're going to better understand and manage your anxieties and stress you really do need to practise regularly. Do you need more reminders? If so, try setting an alarm on your mobile phone, put an eye-catching spot of colour on your watch strap or your memo-board – each time you see it you'll be reminded to check your breathing or to relax. Do you need to make more time for practising? Make a regular 'appointment' with yourself to do this. Could you be more practical? Build practising into your daily routine so that it becomes natural to incorporate it into your day.

It's also important to do the exercises when you feel well and not wait until you feel very nervous. Don't jump in at the deep end. As your skill improves, you'll find it easier and easier to switch to correct breathing or to apply your relaxation skills whenever you feel anxious, but in the early stages of developing your skills, you'll need to try it out when there's the best chance of you succeeding.

'I don't understand the benefit of the exercises when I'm feeling calm. How can I feel the difference between feeling tense and relaxed if I am relaxed in the first place?'

The aim of the exercises is for you to develop the *skill* of controlling your breathing or relaxing at will. This is very different from the experience of feeling relaxed – many people can feel relaxed watching a film or having dinner with friends, for example, but they don't necessarily have the ability to calm and relax themselves if they become over-tense. This is what you're aiming to achieve through the training. As with any skill, you stand a better chance of mastering the basics when you're calm, so that's where the training begins. Even though you are calm, you can still learn to respond to muscular tension by relaxing if you practise the first, lengthy exercise.

'I really don't think I can do this. When I feel nervous I just want to run away.'

As you've already learned, escape is a common response to feeling afraid, so it's quite normal to want to run away rather than stay in a frightening situation and try to relax. The point of learning to control over-breathing and to relax is that it'll give you the confidence to take charge of your nervous feelings so that you don't feel that you have to run away. You'll gain that confidence through practice.

'The sensation of relaxing feels strange, uncomfortable really.'

Learning to relax, particularly if it's a feeling that isn't very familiar to you, can seem quite strange. Some people report feeling odd, not quite themselves, when they first try relaxation. The peculiar feeling is simply because you're not used to it. Some people say that it's so different from their usual way of feeling that it's slightly unsettling, while others describe it as a feeling of letting their guard down, which unnerves them. One benefit of these exercises is that the relaxed feeling will become the more 'normal' feeling, and the anxious one will become something you can quickly dispel. So it's important that you try to carry on and get used to the new feelings, however strange they seem at first. Accept that it will take some practice before it becomes comfortable and, most important, don't worry. Relaxation might be a new feeling, but it's not going to be a bad one.

If you find yourself starting to hyperventilate during the exercise, use controlled breathing to take your breathing back to normal. Prepare yourself by following all the instructions and make sure you're not feeling too hungry, or too full, and that you don't get up too quickly after a relaxation session as your blood pressure may have dropped a little and so you might be a bit light-headed.

'I don't enjoy the tensing sensation during the relaxation exercise.'

Some people say that they feel soreness or cramping during the tensing part of the long exercise. This is usually because they're doing it too vigorously. The experience should never be painful – if it is, ease up a little and perhaps rub the affected muscle if you get cramp. If possible, resume the exercise, but do so gently.

Some people don't like the tensing part of the exercise because it requires them to focus on an unpleasant or even frightening physical sensation. If this is the case for you, practising will soon help you feel less afraid of the sensations because you'll get increasingly good at dealing with them. If you really find that you cannot tolerate the tensing sensation, go on to the shorter exercise and see how you get on with that.

'I get too sleepy.'

Of course, some people relax too well, and fall asleep! If you find yourself dozing off, try not to lie down during the exercise. If you prefer lying down, try holding something (unbreakable!) that would wake you if you nodded off and dropped it. If you have trouble sleeping then make the most of your tendency to drift off to sleep during a relaxation exercise and use it at night when you're going to bed.

'I can't stop thinking about other things.'

You have this in common with almost everyone else so don't *worry* about the thoughts floating in and out of your mind – just accept that this will happen and then simply refocus on your breathing or on the relaxation exercise, whichever you are practising. If you try not to think about something, you're bound to think about it, so just take your mind back to your exercise, rather than trying not to think about something else.

'This is taking for ever.'

Don't lose patience. If it takes some time to master, give it the time. You're probably dealing with something you've had for a long time so it's not going to disappear quickly. You might not feel much benefit when you are first learning to control your breathing or to relax, but the benefits will come with practice. Also, trying too hard is counterproductive. It's a bit like shouting at yourself to relax – we all know that won't work! Be kind to yourself and let the sensations come in their own time and make sure that you're making it easier on yourself by practising, at first, in a quiet, private and comfortable place.

Relaxation Record

When you do your relaxation exercises, write down how you feel before and after and how well it works for you.

Rate your levels of tension on this scale:

0	1	2	3	4	5
Calm, relaxed					As tense as I can imagine

Type of exercise Where and when?	Rating before	Rating after	What I have learnt
Sunday evening on my bed: lengthy relaxation.	4	?	I fell asleep! Although it was nice to have a brief nap that wasn't what I'd hoped for so I will sit down rather than lie down in the future. I wonder if my room was a bit too warm and if I'd have done better if I had not already been tired. I'll try it at a different time tomorrow.
Monday morning alone in the flat, sitting on the sofa: lengthy relaxation.	4	2	It's quite a challenge to go through the whole body without rushing but I was able to do it this time and it paid off. I got rid of a lot of physical tensions and my thoughts were calmer. The benefits lasted for a hour or two as I pottered around the house doing chores, but the tension came back when I went shopping - I realize that I'll have to do the exercise more than once a day.
Wed (two weeks later) - on and off all day. Cued relaxation using getting into my car as my prompt.	3	1	This took about one minute and had a good effect - but I only think that it worked well because I'd already been practising longer relaxation exercises. Getting into my car is an easy 'cue' for me and it's good to be relaxed when I'm driving - less road rage! I'll keep this up.

8

DEVELOPING YOUR COPING SKILLS: TAKING CONTROL OF ANXIOUS THOUGHTS AND IMAGES THROUGH DISTRACTION

Now that you're familiar with ways of tackling the bodily sensations of stress and anxiety, it's time to look at ways of managing the mental aspects – the alarming thoughts and images that race through your mind. Your diary-keeping will have helped you to identify the sort of thinking that either triggers your difficulties or keeps them going. In this chapter you will be introduced to two strategies to help you manage troublesome thinking: distraction and the lengthier process of checking out problem thoughts.

DISTRACTION

This is a relatively simple strategy which you will frequently see people practise for all sorts of reasons. In the dentist's waiting room or in the airport lounge, for example, you might see a man who is getting stuck into a good novel to take his mind off his worries, or a woman with young children playing word games and I-Spy with them to distract them from boredom, or a teenager playing a portable game or listening to music purely for pleasure. The modern world is built for distraction. So how can distraction work for you?

The principle behind distraction is that – although we can do several things at once – we can only truly concentrate on one thing at a time. If that thing is pleasant or soothing, then it is not possible to really focus on alarming thoughts or images. So, if you're thinking about something that makes you feel anxious but can switch your thoughts to something neutral or pleasant, you can distract yourself from your concerns. Your distractions don't have to be exotic. Some great ideas can come from the things you learned at school: listing capital cities, or remembering the plot of a book you had to study, or reciting a school hymn. Use these things as part of your distraction toolkit.

Like other coping techniques described in this book, distraction can work in three ways:

- Preventing the build up of anxiety if you can catch it early.
- Breaking the cycle of anxious thoughts once they've become established.
- Giving you the confidence that *you* can manage your anxiety.

This then means that you can stop avoiding difficult situations and your confidence will grow further. The trick to making distraction work for you is in finding several distractions that really grab your attention. No two people make the same choices because we each have different preferences and interests.

What are good distraction techniques?

The best methods for you will be very specific and will hold *your* attention. If your distraction is too simple, vague or boring, it simply won't engage you. Finding out what does work is often a matter of trial and error, so try out several distractions and see what is most effective.

1. *Keep physically active.* There is really good evidence that physical activity is good for dealing with mild to moderate depression, but getting physical can also help distract you from worrying thoughts. Some people say their minds wander back to their anxieties when doing exercise, but that will be because the task is not mentally absorbing enough for them. So you need to find something that encourages you to think about things *other* than your anxiety, for example, walking through an interesting area, working through a systematic exercise regime, playing a game which involves keeping in mind the rules, or even listening to music or a podcast while you're on the running machine. Physical exercises can also help get rid of the excess adrenaline which, as we saw before, can make you feel uncomfortable. But active distraction doesn't have to be very energetic to be effective – it just has to be mentally absorbing. So, clearing out a cupboard or the garden shed, sorting out books or clothes to give to a charity shop or sorting the contents of your desk drawer, briefcase or handbag can be just as effective as going to the gym. Sometimes doing these things will be more practical and certainly cheaper!

Marci found that going for a walk helped to distract her from her worries:

> *I'm pleased with the way that I'm learning to manage my tension and, in general, I'm much*

calmer. However, things can still stress me out and I find distraction helps me through these times. For example, at work the other day – out of the blue – my boss said that I had to cover for Susie in the afternoon. Susie is brilliant with customers but I'm nervous and I just began to worry and worry about not doing a good enough job. I knew that I was going to have to take over her shift and it was doing me absolutely no good to think about it so much – so I distracted myself. I would have liked to have played a game of squash but that wasn't possible so instead of sitting in the canteen for lunch, I walked across the park and really paid attention to what was around me. It was autumn and I noticed all the different shades of reds and browns in the leaves and the mist hovering over the duck pond. This stopped my thoughts racing – so much so that I could start to think of how I might cope rather than how I wasn't coping.

2. *Keep mentally active*. There are basically three ways of doing this:

- *Simply look at all the things around you* – as Marci did when she was taking her walk.

  Looking at all the things around you simply requires you to pay great attention to your surroundings. Imagine you were sitting on a train. What newspapers are the other commuters reading? What are the headlines? What shoes are they wearing? How many similar styles can you see? If you were walking on the high street, you could ask yourself, 'How many people are using plastic bags?' You could study the details of dresses in shop windows, of pictures and advertisements on the street. If you are on a crowded bus you could listen to someone else's conversation (but be discreet) or music on your personal player. In a supermarket queue you could glance into another customer's trolley and describe their purchases in your head or listen to the in-store music. Essentially, use whatever is around you to take your mind off your anxious thoughts so that you don't get into cycles of unproductive anxiety.

- *Find yourself a mental task* like reciting poems or doing mental arithmetic. The best mental tasks will require enough concentration to keep your mind occupied but not so much that you can't get on with your day-to-day activities. The sorts of things that might engage your attention are tasks like: recalling as many US presidents or British prime ministers as you can; trying to remember which countries were on which sides during the First World War; recalling as many Beatles, Madonna or Lady Gaga songs as possible; remembering the lyrics and tunes of songs; counting backwards, in threes, starting at two hundred; or reciting a poem you had to learn off by heart in school. If words and numbers are not your strength, then think in pictures or music. Think of a real painting or photograph that really struck you, and try to recreate it exactly in your mind, or think of a piece of music that you can recall in detail.

- *Create a soothing image of your own.* You can also make up your own mental pictures, which will take your attention away from stresses. For example, hold in your mind images of your dream holiday, of your dream home, of a favourite activity such as fishing, or an image of your children playing happily. Details will make images more attention grabbing so try to 'see' just where the image is, what the surroundings are like, what the weather is like. Think about what sounds you can hear, what smells there are, who is with you, what you are doing. Try to make it an active image – take a stroll on your dream holiday, walk through each room in your dream home, let your mind follow all the actions involved in fishing, or watch your children play a particular game. The 'richer' your image, the more distracting it will be.

Choose your distraction technique wisely

Before you choose a distraction technique, make sure that it's suitable not only for you but for the situation you're in. For a moment, imagine that you are sitting an exam and your mind is racing with thoughts of failing it. A brief distraction strategy like relaxing your shoulders and counting down from 100 in units of 7 might give you the mental break you need in order to get your thoughts back on the exam question. In that situation, it wouldn't be such a good idea to spend several minutes conjuring up images of your dream holiday as your time is limited and taking a distracting walk would, of course, be out of the question. Another situation might be waiting for a job interview – at such a time it would be better to focus on a soothing image rather than attempt physical exercise in order to control your interview nerves.

Once you have a range of distraction techniques for different occasions, practise them whenever you can. When you are first using distraction, it's possible the scary thoughts will still crop up – just let them pass. Like the other techniques, the more you practise distraction, the more it becomes something that feels quite natural to do.

Constance used distraction to help her with her agoraphobia:

My family doctor always said that she would help me when I felt ready to tackle my agoraphobia. Then I read a self-help book which suggested using distraction to manage some aspects of fear and I thought that I could have a go at that. The first test, for me, was getting to my doctor's clinic, which was about half an hour by bus from where I lived. When I first tried to get there, I felt really panicky and after ten minutes I had to go back home. The next time, I decided to try distraction and I was determined to think about something else, and think about it fully. So I remembered as a child I used to enjoy going to Bible study. I decided I would see if I could say all of the books of the Bible in order, Old and New Testament. And see if I could remember any psalms. I got out of my house, mentally saying, 'Genesis, Exodus, Leviticus' and so on, and felt so distracted I didn't notice my physical state and I didn't get panicky. On the bus, I said a few psalms in my head. The funny thing is, I am no longer religious, but trying to remember these lessons was a good distraction technique and I also remembered how safe and happy I'd felt in those lessons. I managed to get to the clinic and have been able to return several times since, so I now feel confident that I can travel that distance on the bus – my view of myself has really changed for the better. My doctor is very encouraging and she helps me take on increasingly challenging tasks. My progress is slow but steady. In terms of a numerical scale, I would say distraction has brought me down from a 5 out of 5 level of anxiety to 2 out of 5 when I use public transport. This is enormous progress for me and so liberating.

TROUBLESHOOTING: DISTRACTION

'I can't seem to stick with my distracting image.'

Don't get stressed over this as it's very common. Just recognize that it's happened to you and it's time to return to your image. Very importantly, don't try *not* to think about your worries as this will simply bring them to mind more vividly.

'It's just not working for me – my fears and worries are still there.'

Your fears and worries might well still be there, they might not disappear, but by using distraction you might be able to stop them from dominating your thoughts and preventing you from coping with your difficulties. You also might not be choosing the best distraction strategy for you at a certain time. As a rule of thumb, the more anxious you are the better the physical strategies work, and the less anxious you are the more you can engage in the creative mental activities which tend to be more absorbing if you can do them. Also your distraction techniques need to suit *you*: they need to be tailored to *your* interests and preferences. Make sure that they reflect what you're interested in otherwise you might find that they don't really hold your attention.

'I think I might be using distraction to avoid my problem.'

As you can see, distraction can be a simple, portable and effective strategy but you need to look at your use of distraction closely to make sure that it is working *for* you and not *against* you. This is most important.

The aim of distraction is twofold: to help you break out of the cycles of anxiety and worry which only make your fears worse; and to help you get some distance from your problem and clear your head so that you can be more constructive in your thinking. If distraction is working for you, you'll find that you feel more confident that *you* can take charge of your anxiety and you'll find that it gives you the mental break that you need in order to come up with solutions to help you deal with your anxieties.

However, if you find that distraction has become another avoidance strategy which you use to put off facing your fears, then it has begun to work against you and you need to consider using the other techniques in this book.

Constance changed her fundamental belief about herself from 'I can't do . . .' to 'I can do . . .' because distraction helped her learn that she could get around and stay on top of her fears. She developed a more confident view of herself. Viktor, a lecturer with performance anxieties, used distraction in the form of counting but ultimately didn't build his confidence because he had the nagging thought, 'I'm only staying calm before I teach because of my counting routine.' He became almost superstitious about it and grew afraid of taking on challenges unless he used his counting routine. It had become a 'safety behaviour' for him and, if anything, his self-confidence diminished. In order to build confidence, Viktor needed to try to face his fears without using distractions. The strategies in the next section helped him to do this

9

DEVELOPING YOUR COPING SKILLS: TAKING CONTROL OF ANXIOUS THOUGHTS AND IMAGES BY CHECKING THEM OUT

This is the second of the techniques for managing trouble-some thoughts and images. Whereas distraction was about shifting your thinking away from your concerns, now you can develop an additional strategy for tackling them head on. Checking out your anxious thoughts is *not* simply about telling yourself everything is going to be OK; it involves you identifying your troubling thought or image, then standing back and reviewing it critically for exaggerations or misconceptions and then doing a reality check.

CATCHING YOUR WORRYING THOUGHT OR IMAGE

After you've experienced an episode of anxiety, it's not always easy to recall the thoughts or images that triggered or kept it going. You're just *relieved* to be feeling better and may prefer not to examine exactly what happened in detail. But you do need to capture your anxious thoughts so that you can review them and check to see how accurate they are. This is not always easy but whenever you're aware of feeling anxious, ask yourself, 'What is going through my mind?' At first you might conclude 'Blind terror!' but then you need to pause and think what is it *exactly* – what are the words going through your mind? It might be, 'I'm going to have a heart attack,' or 'I think I am going to make a fool of myself.' Or you might think more in images, such as a vivid scene that shows you losing control or something terrible happening.

Keeping a thought diary, a record of what is going through your mind near the time of the anxious episode, is a good way of discovering the words, images or thought patterns that trigger your distress and maintain it. You can use a piece of paper on which you simply jot down your thoughts or you can collect more information and use Diary 2 as your thought diary (see Chapter 6). Alternatively, you can use Diary 3, which is at the end of this chapter, if that appeals to you more. There are lots of variations in diaries – there's no right or wrong one, just the one which works best for you so you might need to try out a few or make up one of your own. Whatever diary you choose, use it to catch what's in your mind when you're feeling anxious or stressed. Alternatively, you could carry a small book and pen around with you, or you can even use electronic devices such as mini voice-recorders or your mobile phone to record what goes through your mind. The most important thing is that it is convenient *for you*. It also needs to be portable so that you have access to it when you're feeling anxious, or very soon afterwards. If you don't catch the thought or image you might lose it.

Even when you are used to keeping a diary, you might not be in a good frame of mind to examine your entries straightaway. This is OK – simply review it when you're feeling calm and fairly neutral. Don't judge yourself. Don't read over it and say, 'Well, that was stupid!' It's not helpful. Instead, be curious: 'I wonder where that came from?', 'Was that a realistic thought?', 'That's interesting, I hadn't realized that I thought that way.'

What you will probably find is that certain themes come up for you, for example: 'I'm looking foolish and everyone notices this', 'I'm ill', 'I will have a panic attack', 'If I don't do this, something bad will happen.'

Once you're familiar with the themes that typically crop up for you, you can begin to review them and think them over.

Isobel started to write down the worrying things that came into her mind:

> *I get nervous about travelling. Keeping a note of what goes through my mind has been eye-opening: no wonder I get nervous when I have thoughts like:*
> - *What if my daughter feels sick and we can't stop?*
> - *What if my son does something dangerous like climbs out of his car seat?*
> - *What if the children just scream and are miserable the whole time?*
> - *What if we get lost, are sick, lose our passports, get mugged . . .*
>
> *It was interesting to see them – they were all questions, and I hadn't realized that my fears were*

> *questions. Seeing them in black and white made them less scary – they were just questions, not facts.*

Once you've identified your anxious thoughts or images, you can stand back as Isobel did and see how you feel about them even before you start to look at them really closely. Isobel noted that her statements were fears and not facts and this helped to calm her. Maybe you will find this, too. If, like Isobel, you find that you ask yourself questions, turn them into statements as these are easier to review than questions. So, for Isobel, the statements would be:

> *My daughter will feel sick and we won't be able to stop the car so she will get really distressed; my son will do something dangerous like climb out of his car seat and get injured; the children will just scream and be miserable the whole time and I won't be able to stand it; we will get lost, become sick, lose our passports, get mugged . . .*

IDENTIFYING EXAGGERATIONS AND MISCONCEPTIONS

When you have recorded your stressful thoughts, first look for patterns of thinking which can exaggerate fears. We looked at these in Chapter 2 and here's a reminder:

1. *Ignoring the positive* – overlooking personal strengths and good experiences and dwelling on the negative aspects of yourself and your life. Isobel probably fails to register the children's good behaviours and all the aspects of the trip which go smoothly.

2. *All or nothing thinking* – viewing things in all or nothing terms and overlooking the possibility that there are degrees of severity: for example: 'the children will just scream and be miserable the whole time'. This sort of thinking can also lead us to hold very high expectations – Isobel might well be setting the standards for children's behaviour far too high and she will be disappointed.

3. *Exaggerating* – magnifying negative or weak aspects, forgetting the positive aspects of a situation and the signs of your strengths. Isobel is overlooking the fact that her daughter has often said that she feels sick and the feeling has passed quite quickly. Exaggerating also includes over-generalizing from one experience – concluding that everything will always be awful because of one thing that has happened in the past.

4. *Selective attention and scanning* – being very sensitive to and searching for the thing you fear (always on the lookout for a threat). Throughout any journey, Isobel was always looking out for the first signs of a problem and she often picked up on things that were not threatening such as the children bickering or her son fidgeting.

5. *Catastrophizing* – anticipating total disaster: for example, 'my son will do something dangerous like climb out of his car seat!'

6. *Jumping to conclusions* – 'mind-reading' and assuming that if you feel something it is fact. 'I feel anxious therefore there must be something to be anxious about.' Isobel always had a feeling of dread when they travelled and so she assumed that things would go badly.

7. *Self-reproach* – blaming and criticizing yourself.

You may find that some of these terms describe very similar ways of thinking. Don't worry about this: it's OK if one of your thoughts fits several terms. The important thing is to realize that the thought is part of the pattern of exaggerated thinking that adds to your fears and worries.

When Isobel did this exercise, she found that she identified quite a lot of extreme thinking which she began to call her 'making a mountain out of a molehill' thinking. Noticing this prompted her to rethink her fears and she was often able to calm herself when she realized: 'There goes my thinking again – it's probably not as bad as I predict.'

DOING A REALITY CHECK

You can do this by taking one anxious statement at a time, and asking yourself questions which will help you get a wider perspective on your concerns. Useful questions are:

- Why does it make sense that I have this concern?
- What is the chance of this worrying thing happening?
- Just what do I think would happen?
- How would I react? How would others react?
- If this thing does happen, how would I respond to it? How would someone else respond to it?

There is more to addressing these questions than you might think as your tone and attitude make a difference. Remember those TV detective interrogations where there's always a 'good cop' and then there's the 'bad cop' who's harsh and critical? You need to be the 'good cop' who is gently encouraging: you need to treat yourself as a caring friend would.

Being the good cop

There are two reasons for taking on this role. First, you're aiming to come up with ideas to give you a wider perspective and the more positive you are, the more relaxed and creative your thinking will be – the 'good cop' approach will help you achieve this. Second, you're aiming to build your confidence and stay calm. A critical inner voice (the 'bad cop') will achieve the opposite. For example, imagine that you are worried that you're going to pass out in church because you did so once a long time ago, on a very hot day. The bad cop might say, 'For goodness sake, get a grip on yourself. That happened ages ago.' Sobering words, not at all soothing or calming. The good cop says, 'Well, you know, it's understandable that you are worried but you will probably be OK, it's not so hot today. But if you do start to feel uncomfortable there are things you can do to calm and distract yourself.'

A more compassionate approach is likely to calm you and keep you in a frame of mind which can help you think around a problem. It could be that you've always used a critical, goading internal voice to get you through things (sometimes we think of this as the 'tough love' voice). If this is the case, then you might find speaking kindly to yourself feels strange and is difficult. You could try to imagine what a really good friend might say as this might give you some kindly inspiration. With practice, you will probably find that you are more able to address yourself in your own (kind) words.

Let's look at Isobel's situation again:

> *I knew I had to do something about my fears. My GP encouraged me to ask myself constructive questions whenever I had these worrying thoughts, almost as if I were another person. I had to consider the 'evidence' that things would go wrong, then imagine the worst-case scenario, and then think how I would deal with it. I thought*

about my worst fear first: my son will do some-
thing dangerous like climb out of his car seat. I
know where this fear came from – I'd seen a film
where it had happened and the child had died and
the image had stayed with me. However, when I
considered the 'evidence' I couldn't think of any
real-life accounts of this happening, my son had
never given me cause to think that he was capa-
ble of unfastening his car seat and I knew that I
was always really careful about fastening him in.
Then I wondered how someone else might handle
this fear and thought that they would probably
reassure themselves that it's normal for mothers
to worry but in this case there really was noth-
ing to fear. To my amazement, I felt better. It was
a whole new way of thinking and I used it to
reconsider all of my fears. Sometimes I discovered
that my fears were founded, like 'We could get
lost' was a possibility, but when I stood back
calmly without being critical of myself, I found
that I was pretty good at planning and problem-
solving. 'Yes,' I thought, 'we could get lost so I'll
make sure that we have all the maps we need and
that I've put the important telephone numbers in
my phone – just in case. No more need to worry!'
It helped not only me but my whole family. We
had our first holiday in ages last summer and
though a few things went wrong, it was nothing
I couldn't cope with. Best of all, I didn't spend
the time leading up to the holiday working myself
up into a state, the way I used to. Now I use the
approach with the children when they are worried
about things.

The approach of standing back and examining alarming thoughts is helpful whether the problem is real or exaggerated – it's a way of being objective about your concerns, not a way of dismissing them. If you still can't spot unhelpful patterns in your thinking ask a close, non-judgemental friend to have a look and to comment on the accuracy of your perceptions and predictions. Remember, you're looking for a bit of objective thinking, not a judgement, so chose your diary-reading friend wisely.

At first it can be difficult to get into the habit of responding to anxious thoughts and images in such a formal way, but with practice it can become natural. Diary 4, which is also at the end of this chapter, can help you develop your skills in reviewing your thinking in a very systematic way. You will see that it has several columns – the first is for you to note down where and when you had the problem thought, the second for you to note down the actual thought or image, then several columns follow which will help you stand back and review your thoughts. You don't have to fill in each column; the purpose of considering them is to help you get a broader perspective.

Let's take a closer look at the useful questions in Diary 4, which will help you complete a reality check of your concerns:

1. *Why does my thinking make sense?* This question will help you work out why you're worried and help you to not feel silly or embarrassed about it. Perhaps some of your fears were borne out in the past or perhaps you have read about a disaster and that's why you have a particular worry: there is usually a reason why certain fears get established in our minds.

2. *What are the 'pros' of my thinking?* Sometimes, there can be *apparent* advantages to anxious thinking – perhaps

you feel that you'll be prepared for the worst by dwelling on the bad things that could happen, or perhaps you have a sort of superstitious belief that if you think something bad, then it won't happen. Understanding the apparent pros of anxious thinking will give you a better idea of why it can be hard to let go of it.

3. *What are the 'cons' of my thinking?* Then consider how your thoughts are unhelpful – in addition to alarming you, of course. For example, they might ruin your social life, limit your work opportunities, set a bad example for your children, prevent you from having enjoyable holidays, etc. This will help you really appreciate the downside of your anxieties and give you more incentive to take the step of overcoming them.

4. *What doesn't fit with my thinking?* Now you are beginning to look at *evidence* – a key concept in Cognitive Behavioural Therapy (CBT) – which will help you rethink your anxious thinking. This is an opportunity to consider all the things which don't fit with your concerns. For example, on reflection, you might realize that the thing you worry about has never actually happened to you or anyone you know; you might recall that you have coped with this particular challenge in the past; you might remember some facts which help you realize that what you fear is unlikely to happen, and so on. This knowledge will help reduce your fears. If it's hard to come up with ideas, ask yourself, 'What would a good friend say in answer to this question?' as this can often help you get a much wider perspective.

5. *What's the worst thing that could happen?* Although this can seem like a daunting task, it's worth considering your worst fear. If you name it then you have identified what have to deal with, if you don't name it the fear remains vague and not easily dealt with. This is particularly so when your thoughts are the 'What if . . . ?' kind

of worries such as Isobel experienced. So often one 'What if . . . ?' just leads to more questions. So, just like Isobel, you need to make a statement about what worries you. When you have worked out what you really fear, then move on to step 6 rather than dwell on it.

6. *How would I cope if the worst thing did happen?* This is a key question which can help you appreciate that you might well be able to manage your fear. If you struggle to come up with ideas, brainstorm either by yourself or by talking to friends and family. You never know: maybe the worst thing did happen to someone you know, and perhaps they got through it and can tell you how. You might find that they say, 'Actually, the anticipation was far worse than the event itself.' Even if they have not experienced the thing you fear, still ask them, 'What would *you* do in this case?' as you might learn from their ideas. Do make sure the person you are asking does not share your particular anxieties, however, as you're looking for alternative views, a different outlook, and some new possibilities or strategies.

Isobel reviewed her fears of travelling:

> *My fear: 'The children will just scream and be miserable the whole time.'*

> 1. Why does my thinking make sense? *The children have screamed and carried on for ages on long journeys. It's made us all very tense and upset and I think that it affects Jon's ability to concentrate on his driving and that's a worry.*

> 2. What are the 'pros' of my thinking? *I suppose I'm prepared for the nightmare if I have thoughts like these.*

3. What are the 'cons' of my thinking? *Although I feel prepared, I'm on edge all of the time, waiting for the next tiff and for Jon to get cross. This means that I don't enjoy the tranquil parts of the journey and I don't relax enough to chat with the children which might actually help ease things. I just wait for the next opportunity to tell them off.*

4. What doesn't fit with my thinking? *To be honest, the children have never screamed and been miserable the* whole *time. In reality they have the odd fifteen minutes of misery before they get distracted by music, the scenery or their own conversations.*

5. What's the worst thing that could happen? *That's easy: the misery would be endless, Jon would get so cross that he wouldn't be able to drive properly and we'd have an accident. I'd never really explored my thoughts before and realized that I'm also concerned about having an accident.*

6. How would I cope if the worst thing did happen? *Well, I could make sure that I did what I could to make it less likely to happen – I could check that the children have enough to entertain them. They all like different things so perhaps I have to put more effort in to my planning. Maybe I could take my own music to listen to so that I could shut out the noise – at least I wouldn't get so bad tempered and I could find out if there is anything which would help Jon concentrate. If we did have an accident, then I guess that we would cope in the same way we have in the past. We would exchange insurance details (so I'll double check that I have copies of all the necessary documents with us) and we would get a replacement vehicle if necessary.*

Ron had fears of being stuck in a tunnel and he also followed the six steps in reviewing his thoughts:

My thoughts: 'Why have we stopped? The train has broken down and we'll be here for ages. It's very warm, I don't have a seat, there's not enough air and I'll have a panic attack.'

1. Why does my thinking make sense? *I got stuck in a tunnel once before. It was only fifteen minutes but the woman next to me started to look pale and clammy and I thought she was going to be sick and this made me very nervous and I had a panic attack. It seemed ages before the train started to move again*

2. What are the 'pros' of my thinking? *I can prepare myself and a panic attack won't take me by surprise.*

3. What are the 'cons' of my thinking? *Rather than helping me ward off a panic attack, my anxious thoughts make me more aware of feeling panicky. I would be better if I didn't dwell on them. I've only ever had the one panic attack – perhaps it was a one-off.*

4. What doesn't fit with my thinking? *Trains often get stuck in the tunnel but not for long. It might only be a few minutes and no one looks as though they're going to be sick – in fact, most*

people look annoyed, not scared – perhaps there's nothing to be afraid of. I've only had one panic attack in a tunnel and the circumstances were different – I have travelled through many tunnels since then and it's always been fine. It's warm in here, but not roasting hot and the windows are open so there must be enough air for us all to be able to breathe comfortably.

5. What's the worst thing that could happen? *The worst thing that could happen is that we do get stuck for some time, and I do start to feel panicky and unwell. I might make a fool of myself if I start to panic.*

6. How would I cope if the worst thing did happen? *Well, this would certainly be a difficult situation for me, but there are things that I can do. I am familiar enough with the feelings of panic to recognize them early and do things to calm myself and remember that I haven't actually had another panic since that first time. Even if I did have another attack, I could ask someone to give up their seat so that I could sit through it – last time people were understanding and helpful, and I got through.*

If, like Isobel and Ron, you've worked through steps 1–6 you will have gathered lots of information about your difficulty and you'll be in a good position to rethink your concerns, to draw new conclusions and develop ideas about coping. If you discover that your worry is realistic, steps 1–6 will have helped you to really define your anxieties and begin the process of problem-solving. Problem-solving is revisited in Chapter 11 and is an invaluable strategy when our concerns are realistic. If your worry isn't a realistic one, you need to make sure that you have drawn a new conclusion which puts your mind at rest – this is addressed in the next section. This can be challenging, but you've done the most demanding part of the work already. Drawing a new conclusion is not about 'spin-doctoring' your situation to make it sound better than it is, but about being *realistic* and constructive.

DRAWING A NEW CONCLUSION

As you saw, Isobel took herself through the six steps. She was then able to look back at her attitude towards herself and her situation and she drew a *believable* new conclusion which helped her deal with her fear:

> *Like any good mother, I'm concerned with safety and the well-being of my family. I know that sometimes I get over-concerned and this makes me lose perspective and stops me from enjoying things. Now I'm aware of what worries me, I can do things to cope. The children are not noisy and miserable all of the time and I can do things to make it more likely that they are distracted and happy and that Jon and I keep calm. Even if the worst thing happened and we had an accident, we have dealt with this in the past and can do so again.*

Similarly, Ron developed a new outlook by going through the six steps:

> *I've had a panic attack in the past so it's no wonder that I'm nervous about having another – that*

makes sense, but I'm pretty certain that I'm under-estimating my ability to cope. I've been managing my anxiety really well and I know that I can recognize and control panicky feelings now. I can read this newspaper and make sure that I keep myself calm. We will probably move very soon now and even if I had a panic attack, unpleasant as they are, I came through before and people are generally kind and understanding.'

TROUBLESHOOTING: TAKING CHARGE OF ANXIOUS THOUGHTS AND IMAGES

'My mind races and I find it really difficult to catch anxious thoughts.'

You're not alone in finding that it can be hard to 'catch' anxious thoughts and images. The first thing to do is relax about it – the tenser you are, the harder it can be to hang on to those thoughts. Then try to record them as soon as you can as it's all too easy to forget the precise thought or image that made you feel anxious. You could keep a piece of paper or a small notebook in your bag or pocket so that you can write down your thoughts quickly or you could make a note of it on your mobile phone.

'It depresses and upsets me to look at what is going on in my mind when I feel anxious.'

Although it would be natural not to want to study your anxious thoughts if you feared that it might be frightening, depressing or embarrassing, most people report that writing down what runs through their minds is helpful. Not only can you see on paper exactly what was going through your mind, but you'll often find that you feel more detached from your thoughts and more able to be objective and rational. Soon you'll be using these notes as a basis for developing a less anxious response: it's a means to a very helpful end.

'It just feels like I'm spin-doctoring myself. I'm saying the words in my head but not really feeling them.'

At first, your new viewpoint might not 'feel' real and it will be hard to hold on to it. It's common to have nagging doubts about your new way of thinking *because* it is a new way of thinking. Your old 'bad cop' voice will butt in from time to time with some critical statement, which might throw you and undermine your confidence. Don't let it get to you as it's quite usual and in time the 'bad cop' will give up and you'll find that you have more confidence in yourself. However, given that it can be such a challenge to believe new conclusions, it's best to write down your new ideas rather than relying on your memory. Then they are there for you to read as many times as you need.

Diary 3

When you feel anxious or scared or stressed, note what goes through your mind.

Rate your levels of distress on this scale:

0	1	2	3	4	5

Not at all scared or stressed
Calm

As scared, worried or stressed as I can imagine being

When this happened and where I was	How I felt (rating)	What was going through my mind: thoughts & images	What I did	How I felt (rating)	What I have learnt
Wednesday, middle of the night: lying in bed.	Worried 5	Lots and lots of worries: What if I don't get the bank loan? I could lose my business. How will I tell Jean? Oh God, the kids – how will they manage if I can't support them?	Lay there until I fell asleep at around 4 a.m.	Worried 5	One frightening thought just leads to another. I start to <u>catastrophize</u>. I <u>ignore the positive and jump to conclusions</u>. Lying in bed worrying doesn't do a thing to help. Funny thing is things never seem so bad in the daytime. I'm not nearly so stressed by those thoughts now. Perhaps I'll remind myself of this next time and see if I can put them to rest by reassuring myself.

Situation	Mood	Thoughts	What happened	Mood after	Response
Sun: getting Molly ready for choir.	Anxious 4	I'm going to have to mix and mingle with the other 'Choir mums' at church. They'll see I'm boring and no one will want to chat with me. I have this picture of myself standing in the corner alone and pathetic. I don't want to go – I am pathetic, aren't I?	Took Molly to choir. Kept my head down. No one spoke to me.	Awful, really down. 4	My head's so full of negative thoughts – all or nothing thinking, jumping to conclusions and self-reproach – it's no wonder I'm nervous and I give up before I even get there. I dread the thought but I think that I'll have to start taking the initiative rather than holding back. If I don't I'll be more scared next time and I'm getting depressed about it. But I need to be able to deal with my worries and my negative thinking first.
Friday: in the pub with friends.	Anxious 3–4	I didn't see the bartender fill my glass – he could have used a dirty one and I could pick up a virus. I could get ill. I could pass it on.	I 'accidentally' spilled my drink and got another.	Fine: 0 for anxiety but I felt silly	Once again I gave into my fears instead of daring to drink from a glass that could have been dirty. Right now I feel such an idiot – but at the time the threat seems so real. I've learnt that I've got two minds – my 'anxious' mind which is prone to catastrophic thinking and my 'sensible' mind – I've got to try to bring my 'sensible' mind into play more often.

Diary 4

When you feel anxious or scared or stressed, note what goes through your mind and then do a reality check by filling in the diary below.

Rate your levels of distress on this scale:

0	1	2	3	4	5

Not at all scared or stressed
Calm

As scared, worried or stressed as I can imagine being

What went through my mind	Why does my thinking make sense?	What are the 'pros' of my thinking?	What are the 'cons' of my thinking?	What doesn't fit with my thinking?	What's the worst thing that could happen?	How would I cope if the worst did happen?	What have I learnt?
Wed night: lots and lots of worries. What if I don't get the bank loan? I could lose my business. How will I	There's a chance that I won't get the loan and it will lead to some real problems.	I won't get caught by surprise.	I get caught up in catastrophic thoughts and worry more and more, and then I can't plan properly.	We've had crises before and I've always managed to pull us through. The family is supportive	The business folds.	We've enough assets to sell off and then we could reinvest. I could go back to being an IT	It's very easy for me to get overwhelmed by catastrophic thoughts at night. The business is under threat – so it's understandable that I worry – but there's a reason-

tell Jean? Oh God, the kids – how will they manage if I can't support them? Rating: worried 5		I can protect myself by not taking risks.	I can't live a normal life.	and strong and the kids are earning now.		consultant as I was before. Jean can always get work as a nurse.	able chance that we'll come through. And even if we don't the family is still strong and I can make a living in other ways. I'll remind myself of this next time I start to worry at night. Rating: worried 1
Friday night: I didn't see the bartender fill my glass – he could have used a dirty one and I could pick up a virus. I could get ill. I could pass it on. Rating: Anxious 3-4	It is possible that the glass has not been washed and it is possible that there are bugs on it.			All my friends drink in pubs without inspecting the glass first and none of them has been ill afterwards.	I get sick and I infect someone else.	I'd keep away from others and take myself off to bed – if I didn't get better I'd phone the doctor sooner rather than later.	Although I see why I have my fears I can also see that I'm really very unlikely to get ill if I relax about drinking in pubs. No one I know has caught something nasty and I won't either – even if I did I know how to look after myself. Rating: Anxious 1-2

10

DEVELOPING YOUR COPING SKILLS: FACING THE FEAR STEP BY STEP

The idea of facing your fears will be daunting – if it weren't you wouldn't be reading this book – but be reassured that it can be tackled in a graded way so that you never have to feel unbearably afraid. You can take a series of steps, *gradually* building up to facing the thing you fear most and, as long as the steps are organized in such a way that you have a good chance of succeeding at each stage, you will steadily build your confidence. Mike overcame his fear of water in this way:

> *I had this swimming instructor back in the early 1970s. I was scared but he just said, 'Nonsense, this is a swimming pool, you can't drown,' and he just chucked me in. I sank like a stone, swallowed loads of water and he had to come in and get me. I had swallowed so much water I was sick in the pool. They had to stop the lesson and afterwards*

the other children made fun of me. I didn't go near water for years after that. Then in my early forties I found a course for adult beginners. I told them the story and explained that I wanted to take things very slowly. I spent two lessons just moving in the water before I felt OK about putting my face in, and then I took another few lessons before I felt confident enough to try to float. In all, it took about ten lessons before I felt comfortable in the water, but each step had involved conquering a little bit more fear and then I found that I could move on to the next step. I wasn't put under any pressure and that worked very well for me and I eventually learnt how to swim. Now I enjoy swimming and even find it a good way to work off stress, which was an unexpected bonus!

In this example you can see how important it was that Mike built on a series of successful experiences, which then increased his confidence.

Gilly has a lift phobia and she can't even contemplate stepping into a lift – however, she could start by looking at a picture of one. This might trigger some anxieties, but at a manageable level. Once this first step felt OK, her next step might involve watching a video clip of someone in a lift, and when she's confident about doing this, her next challenge might be walking in and out of a lift while her friend held the doors open. She then might consider going one stop in this lift with a friend. One by one, this series of slightly more challenging steps would help her to gain confidence that she could use a lift and eventually take one alone. The pacing of the steps would be tailored to what Gilly felt she could manage – bigger steps or faster pacing if she felt more confident and smaller steps or slower pacing if she was unsure of herself.

By breaking down this challenge into a series of steps Gilly would be able to 'bypass' her belief that she could not even contemplate stepping into a lift and she could actually begin facing her fear. Each smaller goal will not only seem achievable but she would get a sense of achievement with each step. This would boost her flagging confidence.

If you have decided that it's time to face your fears, make sure that you are familiar with the strategies in the chapters dealing with bodily sensations of fear and worrying thoughts. You can use these techniques to manage the potentially frightening feelings and thoughts which can come up. This will help you develop your self-confidence.

'TOP TIPS' FOR FACING YOUR FEARS

We might as well start out with the guidelines for good practice, so here they are:

- *Be specific* in describing your ultimate target or goal and in describing each step towards achieving that goal: vague goals and steps are hard to stick to, particularly when you are under stress. Also, it is difficult to give yourself credit for your achievement if it was not clear just what you were meant to achieve.
- *Be realistic* in planning each step: you need to push yourself enough to see progress but not so much that you can't make the step. A useful question to ask is: 'Will this next step stretch me without risking a setback?' Don't try to take on too much too soon and be prepared to be flexible – be prepared to adapt and update your plans according to how you are feeling.

Some days you'll simply have more confidence and energy and you'll be able to take on more.

- *Be creative*: there are many ways in which you can make a step more achievable. For instance, you could go to places that have set off your fears, first of all at quiet times and then build up to busy times; enlist the help of a friend and gradually work towards facing your fear alone; face a less frightening object (e.g. a small kitten) before facing more frightening ones (e.g. a full grown cat); look at pictures or use your imagination before going into a real situation. In this chapter you'll learn about the good guidelines for facing your fears but within these guidelines you can be as creative as you like in order to meet *your* needs.

- *Pace yourself*: you need to get a balance between not feeling too pressured (as this will raise your anxiety levels) and practising regularly enough to see results and build your confidence. Pacing is crucial to the success of 'graded practice' (which means taking it step by step) and it requires some thought. The best person to decide the pace of the steps is you, but you can enlist the help of a friend or a professional if this makes it easier for you to make your decisions.

- *Anticipate setbacks* and understand them: there will be times when things don't go to plan and you don't achieve what you set out to achieve. This is not a 'failure', but an opportunity to reflect on your strengths and needs, and to revise and update your plan. When you have a setback ask yourself: 'Why is this understandable?'; 'What have I learnt?' and 'How can I use this knowledge to make a new plan?' So, if you were trying to overcome your fear of using trains by taking the step of using a small local one, but then you found that you were too scared to leave the platform, rather than assume that you'd 'failed', you could ask yourself the three questions.

Why is this understandable? 'Maybe I took on too much too soon – the station was much busier than I had expected and that raised my anxiety.'

What have I learnt? 'I need a bit more time to get used to the stress of waiting at the station and I need to start my practice at a quieter time.'

How can I use this to make a new plan? 'I can revise my plan to include the task of simply standing on the station and feeling comfortable with that. I'll start at quiet times and work my way up to the rush hour.'

- *Be compassionate towards yourself*: always strive to be kind in your summing up of your performance. Give yourself credit for what you have achieved. Try to *understand* when things don't always go so well. This will help build your self-confidence. You also need to give yourself a bit of an incentive by making your practice as pleasurable as possible. Think about the advantages of what you're doing and think of ways of rewarding yourself. For example, if you were trying to get on a train, you could keep your focus on the end goal, and how much you have to gain, maybe by thinking about how many interesting places you could get to, once you could ride the train. You also need to cheer yourself on every step of the way so you build in a reward each time you progress through a step – you could buy yourself a glossy magazine or some flowers or take some time to go to the cinema. Once you've achieved your goal, mark the occasion by doing something special.
- *Don't put off facing your fear*: doing so can raise your anxieties so bear in mind that the longer you avoid

the thing you fear, the greater the fear you might have to overcome.

CLARIFYING YOUR GOAL OR TARGET

Let's look at Gilly's fear of lifts again. Once she'd decided that she could consider tackling her fears, she came up with a very specific goal: 'To be able to use the glass lift at the front of Smith's department store and to travel from the ground floor to the top – the fifth floor – alone.'

This was a clear goal and Gilly would know when she'd achieved it. If she could take this particular lift in Smith's department store, she knew that she could use virtually all the lifts she needed to use, so it was an excellent 'ultimate' goal.

If you have more than one fear, you'll need to be clear about each of your goals for each of your fears. Gary initially said that his fear was 'a fear of going places', but when he gave it more thought, he actually identified three distinct fears:

1. Flying: I'm afraid of being cooped up and having a panic attack so I'm afraid of all flights, but those lasting over two hours are the worst and I feel more afraid if I'm alone.

2. Motorway driving: I'm scared on all major roads but motorways are worse, especially if they are busy, if it's dark and if I'm alone. I fear that I'll have a panic attack at the wheel.

3. Eating in public: I feel more self-conscious the more fancy the restaurant and the less well I know other guests. It's easier for me if I avoid food which does not need much cutting (so I'm not embarrassed by struggling) or chewing (so I don't risk choking and getting embarrassed that way).

These descriptions of three problems formed the basis for his three goals:

1. *Taking a transatlantic flight by myself so that I can meet my dad and his new wife.*

2. *Driving alone from Stafford to Warwick using the main motorways, alone and at dusk on a working day, when it is quite busy.*

3. *Eating in one of three fancy restaurants in the evening with work guests who I don't know very well. I'll order food which needs to be cut and which is chewy.*

Each goal is described specifically enough for Gary to have a clear idea of what he is aiming for and, like Gilly, he is sure that if he can reach these targets, he'll be pretty much able to 'go places' with confidence. You need to have the same standards – make your goals precise and make sure that they will enable you to do the things that you want to do. When you work out your goal list, make sure that it isn't unnecessarily long: just stick to those goals that are important to you and your quality of life. These are the things you'll be most motivated to tackle. If one of your phobias is, for example, lions and you don't live in the wilderness and are not fond of zoos or safari holidays and you can tolerate seeing images of lions, then overcoming your fear of them is not going to have a great impact on the quality of your life. You might do better tackling a fear that actually does interfere with your enjoyment of life and your freedom to do what you want to.

Try this for yourself and write down your targets in the space below.

My goals or targets:

DEVISING YOUR STEP-BY-STEP APPROACH

Once you've thought about your goal, you might find that you already have ideas about how you can achieve it. Everyone's fear is different and in order to plan how best to face *your* fear, you'll need to understand the *precise* nature of it.

Let's revisit Gilly – in order to devise her step-by-step plan to achieve her goal, she would need to ask herself questions like:

- Is there any lift I can tolerate right now?
- Which lifts make me feel more or less anxious?
- Is it better if I'm alone or with someone?

- Does it make a difference where I am, or what time of day it is?
- What exactly am I afraid of – the lift falling down or it getting stuck?
- What could I manage right now?

When she had considered just what made it easier or harder for her to use lifts, she recognized that:

> *Crowded lifts are worse than empty ones for me.*
>
> *Old lifts are scarier than modern, well-maintained lifts.*
>
> *Open or glass-sided lifts are worse than enclosed lifts: it's more about the height than the confinement.*
>
> *It's better if I am with a friend.*
>
> *It's better if we are not stopping at every floor – that just prolongs the agony.*
>
> *I could imagine standing in a lift which is not moving.*

Now she understood just what made her feel most afraid and what she could tolerate, she was able to plan her first step.

> My first step: *I could probably manage to go one flight in a large, enclosed lift, from basement to ground floor. I could do this in Smith's department store at a very quiet time, like first thing on Sunday morning, with my friend Anke to give me support.*

This was Gilly's starting point and from there she went on to develop her ideas – which she could always adapt later:

I will then try to work my way up to the top floor – still at a quiet time and with Anke to help. When we get to the top I will treat us in the café. Once I can get to the top at a quiet time, I'll ask Anke if she'll come with me in the afternoon when it's busier and we'll aim to get to the top again. When we do, I'll treat us to a cream tea. Then I think that I'll be ready to go it alone – at first on Sunday morning but gradually I'll tackle the lifts at busier times. Each time I succeed at a step I'll return to the cosmetics department and buy myself something as a reward.

Marcia had a different goal, she wanted to be able to eat freely at restaurants in her home town, without feeling too anxious – here she pinpoints the exact nature of her fear of eating in public.

It is worse for me if the restaurant is busy as I feel self-conscious as well as afraid of being sick.

It's also worse if I can't see the kitchen – so I like restaurants with open kitchens and I like to sit near them.

I also like to sit near the cloakroom in case I am ill.

It doesn't matter how fancy the place is, just how clean it looks, and it must have good lighting as I don't trust dark places to be hygienic.

It's always easier for me if I eat vegetarian as I don't think that you can get food poisoning so easily.

It's always easier with a friend as they keep me distracted and relaxed.

My first step: *I could probably eat at several of the 'clean', well-lit restaurants in the city as long as the kitchen was visible, as long as I ate vegetarian and as long as I was with a good friend. Later I might be able to use one of the less well lit eating places and I might be able to eat meat.*

By considering her fear in more detail, Marcia was able to tailor the first step to her strengths which would make it very possible that she would succeed. She didn't have such specific ideas for the next few steps as Gilly had, but she had a good idea about where she would take things and this is enough to start with. After she has completed her first step she'll have an even clearer idea of her strengths and she can build on this to create a list of steps to take her to her target or goal.

Grading your tasks

If you have analysed your fears and worked out your starting point, you can move on to making the list of *achievable* steps which will link what you can do right now to your goal. You might ask yourself, 'Well how can I know if it is achievable if I haven't done it?' Good question. You are going to have to speculate a little and you'll need to be prepared to 'fine-tune' your list as you make progress, but for now aim for steps which will stretch you, yet do seem achievable. While you don't want to set yourself up for failure by taking on something too difficult, you do want to do something that gives you the chance to practise coping with your anxiety. A good question to ask yourself when making your list is, 'Can I imagine doing this with a bit of effort?' If you answer 'No' then make the task a bit easier.

You know your strengths and preferences better than

anyone so you'll have a good idea of what would make it easier. Perhaps a different time of the day? A friend's support? Fewer people? More distraction? But keep in mind that you're aiming to push yourself enough to see progress and that you're aiming to steadily increase the difficulty of your tasks. You will have to move out of your comfort zone.

Getting this balance can be quite difficult so don't be hard on yourself if it takes a trial or two and consider asking a friend or professional for help in planning your tasks.

When you have defined your goals, decide which is either most urgent or easiest for you to tackle and focus *just on this*. Remember, even if you are full of gusto and motivation, tackle one target at a time. You don't want to give yourself so many challenges that you risk being overwhelmed.

Gary's starting points were:

> 1. *I can tolerate being on a short-haul flight with my wife or a colleague.*
>
> 2. *I can use the local ring road which is a dual carriageway and I can use this in rush hours.*
>
> 3. *I can eat with my family in a moderately fancy restaurant (e.g. Romano's) and I can eat pretty much anything when I'm with them.*

He decided that his most pressing challenge was motorway driving as his inability to travel by car was interfering with his ability to do his job, so he decided to work on that first. You'll see just how detailed his plan was – this is what you need to be aiming for, too.

> *Goal: Driving alone from Stafford to Warwick using the main motorways, alone and at dusk on a working day, when it is quite busy.*

Step 1: Driving on the familiar, local ring road (dual carriageway) when it is quiet.

Step 2: Driving on the familiar, local ring road (dual carriageway) during the rush hour as it's getting dark.

Step 3: Driving on the city ring road, which is busier and less familiar, on a Sunday morning when it's quiet.

Step 4: Driving on the city ring road on Saturday afternoon when it's busy.

Step 5: Driving on the city ring road in the rush hour at dusk.

Step 6: Driving from junction 13 to junction 14 of the motorway with Philip (to give me a bit of confidence).

Step 7: Driving from junction 13 to junction 14 of the motorway alone.

Step 8: Driving from junction 13 to junction 15 of the motorway alone.

Step 9: Driving from Stafford to Warwick with Philip on a quiet day (and returning on the same day).

Step 10: Driving from Stafford to Warwick (return) with Philip at a busy time.

Step 11: Driving myself to Warwick and making the return journey alone at 5 p.m. when it's busy and beginning to get dark.

Gary had the good idea of making things easier for himself by relaxing before each journey, by using the quieter toll road for part of the journey and by having some soothing music in the background when he was alone. He also made the task more enjoyable by making sure that he celebrated his achievements – for example, he and Philip planned to go to a motor show on one of their journeys and a football match on another.

For Gary, it is clear that the amount of traffic, the time of day, the length of the journey and whether or not he is alone are all challenging aspects of the task, so it was sensible that he introduced changes one at a time rather than several aspects at once. You should aim to do the same: only change only one aspect of the task at a time. Welcome each task as a step towards your goal, and also as an opportunity to practise your coping skills.

Try breaking down your target into small, specific tasks.

My goal/target and tasks

My goal or target:

My tasks:

1.

2.

3.

4.

5.

6.

and so on.

PRACTISING

Now it's time for the practical part of facing your fear. You'll need to take on each step one at a time. It is best to keep practising a particular step until you can manage it without difficulty as the plan is to feel comfortable before you move on to the next step. This way you increase your chances of succeeding and you build your confidence. However, if one practice session doesn't go so well, give yourself a pat on the back for having a go, try to understand why it didn't work out this time and, if necessary, revise your plans. Then try again.

To be effective, the practice should be:

• Regular
• Rewarding
• Repeated

This means that you need to do the following:

• Make sure that your plans fit it in with your lifestyle.
• Regularly make time for your practice.
• Reward yourself for your successes (a mental pat on the back will do, it doesn't have to be material).
• Be gentle and kind to yourself when it doesn't go well.
• Repeat each step until it feels easy for you.

Now we'll follow Gary's progress and you'll see that over-coming his fear took time and planning – this is often the case, so make sure you are realistic about the time and effort involved when you make your own plans. Gary put a date in his diary to begin his practice and he found that the first step was so easy for him that later in the afternoon he took on step 2. With hindsight, step 1 might have been too simple, but it is better to err in that direction and ensure success, rather than risk taking on too much. All this had gone so smoothly that he decided to take on step 3 the following Sunday, and in the meantime continue to practise step 2 so that he kept building his confidence. He was looking forward to trying out a more challenging task and disappointed when it proved more stressful than he'd expected. Gary managed to get round the city ring road but he was very nervous and began to worry that he might panic.

He took the right approach to this disappointment: he was not hard on himself and at home he looked back on his experience and realized that he would have been calmer if he been more certain of the road layout – *he learnt from the setback*. He studied a map of the area and he asked his wife to drive him round the ring road a few times so that he got a better feel for it. The following Sunday he tried again and it went much more smoothly. He had learnt the importance of preparation. He also learnt that it was impractical to have to wait a week before he could practise again so he revised his plan and replaced steps 4 and 5, so it gave him more options and more chances to practise. The new steps were:

Step 4: Diving at a quiet time before dark.
Step 5: Driving at a busy time before dark.

He continued to practise regularly and soon reached step 6, where he drove on the motorway with Philip. He discovered that he could combine steps 7 and 8 and he drove for two junctions alone. Buoyed up by this success, Gary and Philip set out to make the journey from Stafford to Warwick. This proved too much of a challenge – Gary hadn't anticipated that the motorway junctions would be quite so complicated and he began to panic half-way there. They pulled into a service station and talked about what was happening and considered their options. They could:

- Return to Stafford with Philip driving.
- Return with Gary driving.
- Continue to Warwick with Philip driving.
- Continue to Warwick with Gary driving.

Feeling calmed by the break, Gary chose to continue the journey himself but with the options of taking another break if necessary or handing the driving over to Philip. The important lesson that he learnt from this setback was *have back-up plans.*

Gary needed to repeat this journey with another driver several times in order to get ready for a solo outing and Philip simply was not available as often as Gary needed him. Therefore, Gary revised his plans again. He asked another friend and his brother to become involved. This took some courage on Gary's part as he was rather embarrassed by his fears, but he felt that the benefits of continuing his practice would outweigh the cost of revealing his secret. In this way he was able to complete his tasks and achieve his target. When asked what he had learned from his experience, he said that he now realized the importance of:

- Good planning.
- Learning from setbacks.
- Flexibility.
- Practice, practice, practice.

TROUBLESHOOTING: GRADED PRACTICE

'This idea looks great on paper. I just don't think I have the courage to do it in real life.'

Of course your plan will look challenging – it's about facing something that you find frightening. However, you can do this if:

- The steps are well thought through and designed to give you the best chance of success – make sure your steps build on each other.
- You anticipate there will be times when things don't go according to plan and you're prepared to learn from this and revise your ideas, maybe breaking down a challenge into smaller steps.
- You are compassionate and understanding so that you're not too hard on yourself. Don't force yourself to take on too much and don't criticize yourself – instead recognize your achievements and reward yourself if you can.
- You feel supported – maybe a friend or professional can be involved in your plans to face your fears.

'It's all gone horribly wrong – it's hopeless!'

You will have setbacks from time to time – everyone does. Keep notes of what happens during your practice and then you might be able to see why certain tasks were harder than others. Be curious and compassionate rather than critical and try to understand why things didn't go well – perhaps you were already stressed, perhaps you were tired or under the weather or perhaps you took on too much. You won't always be able to identify what went wrong and, if you can't, rather than worry about this, let it go and try again.

Watch out for negative thinking, which can set you back even further: 'It's all gone horribly wrong – it's hopeless!' is an example of the sort of extreme thinking that could sap anyone's confidence.

'This idea looked great on paper but it didn't work in real life.'

Your plans must fit in with your lifestyle and your resources. If you have a full-time job and an inflexible boss, then planning activities during the working day would not be wise. If you have children, then you'll have to consider what childcare you have and when – and then plan around this. If you have limited income you need to plan within the constraints of your budget – taking repeated trips on public transport might be a good idea in theory but not one which is affordable. If the rewards which you promised yourself reflect what you think you ought to enjoy rather than what you do enjoy, then they won't be such a good incentive to persist with your practice. It's really worth investing time in the planning stage as this will stop you from wasting time later.

11

DEVELOPING YOUR COPING SKILLS: PROBLEM-SOLVING

We all know someone who is good in a crisis. They remain capable, calm, and seem to have some sort of knack or method of handling any problem that arises. Wouldn't it be great to be like that? Can someone with a history of anxiety problems become a person like that? Perhaps not naturally, but by learning the steps involved in problem-solving it is achievable. In addition, changing your way of thinking and learning how to remain calm (see Chapters 8 and 9 on this), or modelling yourself on a person who's very good at solving problems, can further enhance your ability to solve problems that would otherwise make you anxious.

You've just learnt about graded practice as a way of managing fears and anxieties – what can problem-solving add? Graded practice involves using a structured plan which assumes that you have a certain amount of time available to you to practise and pace yourself. Sometimes this isn't practical because the thing you fear or find stressful is imminent and you don't have time to follow a step-by-step approach. You might have a holiday, or a big family gathering, or a work presentation coming up and you might not be able to devise a graded practice programme in time for the event. You'll need to come up with a 'plan B' quite quickly. This is where problem-solving comes in. It's a useful approach for organizing and focusing your thinking so that you can come up with several solutions quite quickly. This means that you don't have to fall back on avoidance.

There are seven important but clear steps in problem-solving:

1. Identify the problem

2. Brainstorm

3. Review your solutions

4. Combine and order your ideas

5. Plan

6. Put solutions into action

7. Assess progress

We'll look at each of the steps in more detail so that you get an idea of how this can work for you. We'll use the example of Monica who was very anxious because she had to give a presentation at work.

1. IDENTIFY THE PROBLEM

As in planning graded practice, you need to be specific about the task ahead, don't confuse several tasks and always take one problem at a time. When possible, distinguish between the different aspects of your difficulties and separate them out into a collection of more manageable tasks. Then make a plan for each. Let's see how this worked for Monica.

> *I have to give a presentation at work next week. I have to know what I'm talking about and not show that I am nervous. I'll be in a small, poorly ventilated meeting room for at least an hour. What if it goes wrong? What if they don't like my ideas?*

This describes her difficulties but, for problem-solving to be effective, she needed to be more specific. She needed to consider precisely:

- What is going to happen?
- When will this happen?
- Who is involved?

She also needed to address her worries rather than holding worrying questions in her mind. She came up with:

> The task: *I have to give a thirty-minute presentation to fifteen colleagues at work next Thursday. I have to know my subject by then and be prepared to answer questions. I will be in a small, poorly ventilated meeting room for at least an hour.*

> My fears: *I hate being the focus of attention. I worry that I'll forget what I have to say or not be able to answer questions, and the audience will realize that I'm stupid and incapable. I'm afraid that the confines of the room and the lack of fresh air, combined with my presentation fears, will trigger a panic attack.*

Once she had defined her task and her fears, she could see that there were two aspects to it:

a. Preparing herself and feeling confident about presenting her topic on the day.
b. Dealing with her fears of panicking.

Monica was confident that she knew how to prepare her presentation and she knew that rehearsing it with a friend would help manage her performance fears, so she decided to prioritize the second issue (panicking in the confined space) for problem-solving.

2. BRAINSTORM

This means thinking of as many solutions as possible (even if they seem odd) *without pausing to judge them*. It's important to simply write down ideas without questioning them – this way you will not interrupt your flow of thoughts and sometimes the 'odd' solutions turn out to be quite creative and helpful, so we want to include them. If it helps, imagine yourself in the shoes of someone you know who is good at problem-solving and try to think in the creative way he or she might. Write down the solutions so that you don't forget them.

Monica's list of options looked like this:

- *Ask my boss to move the meeting to a larger, more airy room.*
- *Ask Jake to co-present so that he could take over if necessary.*
- *Ring in sick/leave saying that I feel sick.*

- *Ask my boss to change the meeting to a telephone conference.*
- *Wear cool, comfortable clothes.*
- *Have a cool drink to hand.*
- *Allow myself to take a break if I feel panicky.*
- *Ask the audience members to read the handouts themselves if I get flustered.*
- *Incorporate small group discussions into the presentation so that I have the odd break to compose myself, if necessary.*
- *Imagine that the people in the audience are all my good friends who wish me well.*
- *Ask Carol what she would do – get some more ideas.*
- *Relax before the meeting.*
- *Rehearse my presentation so that I'm at least confident about that.*
- *Relax during the meeting – keep a relaxed posture and smooth breathing.*
- *Ask my boss to move the time of the meeting to the morning when I tend to cope better anyway.*
- *Remind myself that I've been here before and coped.*

3. REVIEW YOUR SOLUTIONS/
4. COMBINE AND ORDER YOUR IDEAS

Now is the time to look at your ideas more critically. Amongst them there will be some you can use, some that should be rejected outright and some that you might hang on to as 'back-up' plans which you would only use if you really had to. When Monica did this she came up with the following:

Reject these ideas:

- *Ask my boss to change the meeting to a telephone conference: no point as we work in the same building.*
- *Ask my boss to move the time of the meeting to the morning when I tend to cope better anyway: impossible to shift the time.*

Hang on to these ideas (best first):

a) *Ask my boss to move the meeting to a larger, more airy room – the sooner I do this the better.*
b) *Ask Carol what she would do – get some more ideas.*
c) *Relax before the meeting – I know lots of ways of doing this.*
d) *Incorporate small group discussions into the presentation so that I have the odd break to compose myself, if necessary – this is good practice anyway.*
e) *Rehearse my presentation so that I'm at least confident about that – again this is just good practice and I would do it anyway.*
f) *Relax during the meeting – keep a relaxed posture and smooth breathing.*
g) *Wear cool, comfortable clothes.*
h) *Imagine that the people in the audience are all my good friends who wish me well.*
i) *Ask Jake to co-present so that he could take over if necessary.*

j) Ask the audience members to read the hand-outs themselves if I get flustered.

k) Allow myself to take a break if I feel panicky.

Back-up ideas:

- *Have a cool drink to hand (I used to sip water as a safety behaviour, so I don't want to fall back on this unless it's absolutely unavoidable).*
- *Ring in sick/leave saying that I feel sick (although this is avoidance and really the 'worst-case scenario' option, having it there and knowing that I have a way out gives me some comfort – and actually makes me prepared to take on the challenge).*

Some ideas can be combined to make them more effective. For example, combining relaxing *and* using distraction before an event, or combining relaxation with writing out a detailed coping plan.

As is often the case, Monica discovered that several of her ideas combined well and she decided to carry out a) to e) before the meeting and to carry out f) to h) during the meeting. She felt that with this preparation, she'd probably be able to cope but she had ideas i), j) and k) as reserve plans and if things got really bad she had two 'back-up' plans.

If you follow a similar plan, you will be able to create a set of ideas to help you resolve your problem.

5. PLAN

Now you can take your first solution and consider carefully

how you will put it into action: What needs to be done? How? When? With whom? Where? What preparatory work needs to be done? Again, you had some practice in being very specific in planning in the previous chapter, so this might seem more familiar by now.

When Marcia considered idea c) (Relaxing before the meeting) she thought it through carefully and reflected on what she could do to increase the chances of relaxation helping her. She then made a plan to relax every evening before going to bed and each morning on rising so that she really revived her relaxation skills. She also planned to take time alone, in the library, before the presentation to simply relax and she planned to take along her MP3 player so that she could listen to a soothing piece of music to help her. When thinking in more detail about idea i) (asking Jake to step in if necessary) she rehearsed what she would say to him, explaining her needs and the advantages to him of getting more of an active profile in the department. She contacted him as far in advance of the presentation as possible, so as to give him time to think about her proposal. She also ring-fenced time she could spend with him in preparing the presentation. He was very pleased to be asked and willingly agreed to help out.

6. PUT SOLUTIONS INTO ACTION

Once you've planned and prepared, it's time to try out your best solution. In Monica's case, she began by immediately asking her boss if the venue could be changed – unfortunately this was not possible. A further disappointment was that Carol was visiting her sick mother for a few days and Monica didn't want to bother her. However, she wasn't too distressed by this as she had come up with her own good ideas for preparing herself for and coping with the presentation. She simply put her other ideas into action. On the day, she had prepared well for the presentation, was feeling confident about her knowledge of the subject, was reasonably relaxed and was optimistic that she could tackle this challenge.

All went quite well until she began to cough a few minutes before the end and she couldn't stop. It wasn't nerves, it was just bad luck. In the past this would have sent her into a panic, but she had already prepared the option of Jake stepping in for her and she had already thought about the possibility of leaving the room if necessary, so, she calmly gestured to Jake to take over and she left the room to get some water. Rather than feeling afraid or a failure, she congratulated herself on being so well prepared. A minute or two later she returned and was composed enough to answer questions from the audience.

7. ASSESS PROGRESS

Always ask yourself: 'How did it go?' It's important to reflect on how things are going both during your challenging task and afterwards. During the task keep your eye on things so that you can identify potential problems early and bring in a new solution if you have to (as Monica did). Afterwards, it's always helpful to look back and ask yourself: 'What have I learnt from this? What has the experience taught me about my strengths and needs?' Perhaps you learnt that you were able to resist checking the light switches and nothing bad happened; or that you have got the nerve to visit the reptile house at the zoo; or that you need to be less ambitious next time; or that taking on a challenge when you feel ill means that you will struggle.

Remember that if something did not go well that you have not failed: you have just learnt more about your needs. Be understanding.

Monica felt that she had learnt that she was capable in her work and, although nervous about performing, she could do this, too. She also learnt the value of preparing herself and asking others for help. With hindsight, she wouldn't deprive herself of water if she gave another presentation as, after twenty minutes, it's normal for a person's throat to get dry, but she would not sip the water constantly as she recalled this used to be one of her unhelpful coping strategies which sapped her confidence.

In summary, if your solution works, that's great but if it's not working for you go back to your list (step 4) and take your next solution (make sure that you have planned how to put it into action). If this solution doesn't work for you, there's no need to panic because you can return to step 4 again – as often as you need to. If you have made a long list at step 4, you will have lots of options to try.

TROUBLESHOOTING: PROBLEM-SOLVING

'This all takes too long.'

If following through the seven problem-solving steps seems rather long-winded, keep in mind that it's a good investment of time and by the end of the exercise you'll have a whole list of possible solutions so you can relax a little knowing that if the first one doesn't work you have several more to try. This gives you alternatives to avoidance and this, in turn, will give you the chance to build your confidence. Also, remember that you don't need to spend

too long on the brainstorming. Quickly write down possible solutions – however odd they might seem – and don't
spend any time evaluating them: if an idea comes into your
head, capture it and move on.

'It's just not working for me.'

The success of the problem-solving approach depends on
sound planning. Remember that you need to have worked
out several back-up plans so that if your first choice does
not work, you can return to step 4 and choose another
option. It's vital that you do this preparation when you're
feeling calm, and not in the throes of panic when it is hard
to come up with ideas and make good plans.

*'It must be a bad thing to include unhelpful solutions
such as avoidance or leaving the room.'*

The goal of problem-solving is to help you deal with a challenge as best you can and although avoidance or escape are
not good long-term strategies it is OK to have them on your
solution list *as a final resort*. Knowing that *if all else fails*
you can leave the room might just give you the courage to
take on the challenge (as it did for Monica). If you discover
that you've overestimated what you could achieve on this
occasion and that the time is not right for you to tackle a
problem head on (and this will happen from time to time)
then you can fall back on your final resort, knowing that
you tried other solutions before turning to the one that is
not so helpful in the long term. You can then accept that
you gave the challenge your best shot and you can move
on. If you work through the exercises in this book, you'll
build up your range of coping skills and eventually you
will be relying on 'last resort' solutions less and less, if at

all. There will be times when you have to cut yourself some slack and, if you use an emergency measure, this doesn't mean that you have failed. It just means you weren't ready or rehearsed enough to try the longer term strategy or that the circumstances were just not right for you.

12

IN IT FOR THE LONG HAUL: STAYING CALM AND COPING WITH SETBACKS

Coping in the long term doesn't mean banishing anxiety forever, but you will learn to manage it and to live with it. It would be strange (and unhelpful) never to experience anxiety again – after all, it's the normal and vital response to threat. What you *can* expect is to have fewer experiences of anxiety and to reduce the effect it has on your life. You can look forward to developing the confidence that, whatever life throws at you, you'll be able to handle it. However, this doesn't mean that you won't, occasionally, experience rather longer episodes of anxiety or setbacks.

COPING WITH SETBACKS

How you react to setbacks will have a significant impact on your progress. It always helps to treat yourself with kindness and understanding – as you would a friend. If you beat yourself up – 'Here we go again, another thing that didn't work, another failure!' – you might find it really difficult to hold on to your optimism and self-confidence. Research on setbacks shows that if you're compassionate towards yourself and accept that this is just a lapse and that *setbacks are opportunities for us to learn more about our strengths and needs*, then you'll feel less demoralized and you'll be able to take something useful from the experience. Of course, it can be upsetting when you lapse but nonetheless, try to accept it, learn from it and don't agonize over it. Accept how you feel but move on and think productively: 'How can I turn this setback to my advantage?'

It's so important that it's worth repeating that you should always ask yourself:

- *Why didn't it go smoothly?* Were you already stressed? Were you feeling ill or unwell? Was the task different from what you had expected? Were you prepared enough?

- *What have I learnt from this?* Perhaps you now realize that anyone might struggle given so much stress to deal with or given that unforeseen issues arose, for example.

- *Knowing this, what will I do differently in the future?* Perhaps you would now check out the situations more thoroughly or not take on such a big challenge when you had other worries to deal with.

This approach will really help you continue to make progress.

KEEPING UP YOUR PRACTICE

Practising your strategies will also help you make progress. Just as with physical exercise, our stamina and strength diminishes if we don't exercise – we run the risk of our anxiety management strategies not being so effective if we neglect them.

It took Nadia quite some time before she saw that the coping techniques she learned were not just for pulling out on an anxious day, but something she had to build into her lifestyle and make a part of her mindset:

> Now that I'm managing my fears and stress better, I realize that this new way of thinking, feeling and being has to be for life. If I want to be a person who does not suffer with anxiety, I need to keep on top of it with the techniques I've learned. I didn't start dealing with my anxieties until I was thirty-five, and I had been having anxiety attacks for seventeen years, so I didn't expect it was something that was going to change overnight or change for good once I'd learned the techniques. I would still say I am prone or susceptible to anxiety, but that I am so much better at managing it. I will never be a person other people describe as laid-back or chilled, but I think I am a person whose life is not ruled by fears. It's like physical exercise – some people get away with doing very little and they still stay slim and fit, others have to work at it. It's very much the same with what goes on in your mind – some of us have to work at keeping it in shape. If I want to be a person whose life is not ruled or ruined by anxiety, I have to work at it. I try not to think of it as a chore, though – more as a ticket to freedom from fear.

PREPARING FOR FUTURE CHALLENGES

Even though you're probably feeling more in control of your fears and anxieties right now and you might be doing things which seemed impossible before, there will still be challenges in the future. Some of these might come about because life simply presents us with difficulties from time to time, or they might arise because you're now more able to take on new things and tackle new challenges, so you're stretching yourself more. Whatever the reason, you can begin to do some 'troubleshooting' to minimize the impact that stressful situations will have on you.

First you need to think about what your future challenges might be and when you might be most vulnerable to stress. While it's not a good idea – in fact it's a terrible idea – to dwell on everything that can or might go wrong in the future, it's wise to take a realistic view of what might trouble you. This will put you in a position of being able to prepare yourself. Your list of potential difficulties might include situations such as: 'Travelling to Frank's wedding which is a four-hour drive from home', 'Taking an underground train for more than seven stops', 'Keeping my stress under control when I've a lot on at work', 'Managing my worries when I'm feeling tired or unwell'.

Once you've predicted the situations that are likely to be stressful for you, you can make a plan for each challenge. Always think about how you'll relax before the event, and what strategies you'll use when you face it. Consider which coping techniques work best for you in certain situations. Thinking about difficult times doesn't mean you're not coping, it just means that you are doing what you can to be prepared. Once you have worked out when things might be hard you can:

- Try to change a situation to make it easier, for example by spending extra time on planning and problem-solving, getting in some graded practice if that's possible, or finding time for extra relaxation practice.
- Have a realistic and caring attitude, for example by recognizing that you might not enjoy a difficult trip but still giving yourself credit for making it; setting yourself a less taxing goal if you're unwell or feeling stressed; being compassionate in the face of a setback.
- Think what has worked for you so far and make sure that you can still use these strategies – keep up your practice and have ways of reminding yourself what to do. You might find it helpful to carry a small book around with you, or even this book, containing ideas for coping when you are stressed. Some people find it useful to have copies of diaries, descriptions of their most effective coping strategies or reminders of sooth- ing images in the form of pictures for handy reference. Something small, portable and possibly without a title might be best to read in public. Some people fill their mobile phones with relaxing music, helpful notes and soothing pictures – and this is very discreet and very portable.
- Be flexible and have back-up plans. None of us can accurately predict just what will happen in a difficult situation so try to develop a few ideas about dealing with different scenarios.

James managed to beat his fears and worries despite having a setback:

> *I had a fear of flying. It was never just about the flight itself, but I would worry about getting to*

the airport, the crowds, the queues, and then the flight, the confinement, the potential bumps and a feeling of not being able to escape. Through graded practice and relaxation exercises, I had managed to get to the airport. Next I'd been able to go on a short-haul flight, and eventually, a seven-hour flight to from London to New York. Since then, I've been on three return journeys to Europe from the UK, the longest being about four hours. I managed these quite well and even remained calm on one flight where the person next to me was ill the whole time. A few years ago, that would have been unthinkable for me, so I've done really well and I'm pleased with my progress.

Not long ago, I booked another flight to New York and found myself getting nervous beforehand but I tried to put this out of my mind. When I got to the airport I saw that the terminal had changed. It was much nicer and more spacious, but it was not what I expected and this increased my anxiety and the flight itself was difficult. I had peaks of anxiety, and they would go down for a bit, but overall, I felt very nervous and uncomfortable, and upset that I wasn't coping as well as I imagined I would. I had a couple of alcoholic drinks and this seemed to help for a bit, but then I felt dehydrated and ill. Finally, immigration in New York was a nightmare. The queue was at least an hour long and everybody was fed up and this made me more nervous. I had to find a guard and tell him I wasn't feeling well, and he let me jump the queue.

I made sure that I made time to think about this experience and to use what I'd learnt to plan my return journey. I realized that it was no wonder that I'd had this setback: I was out of practice and I had not prepared myself for such a long flight and the complicated checking-in and immigration procedure. I think that I tried to ignore the fact that there might be difficulties. I also got caught up in an unhelpful cycle: I became disappointed with myself, which made me less confident and less able to cope, which then increased my disappointment. On top of it all I went for the 'quick fix' of alcoholic drinks, which always makes me feel worse in the long term. I could see where I'd gone wrong and was determined use this knowledge to plan my return trip – and to do this in good time. So, I practised my relaxation exercises and then I could better calm myself when I needed to (rather than relying on alcohol) and I had some soothing music and a novel with me so that I always had a distraction if I felt that I was getting wound up whilst waiting around. Finally, I remembered not to be critical of myself but instead understand why I might struggle with some things and still give myself credit for taking on the challenge. The return flight was a much better experience – thanks to my planning there were no nasty surprises and I was able to use my coping strategies to keep on top of my anxieties. I even managed to sleep for an hour or two by using a lengthy relaxation exercise. What I learnt was being prepared and being compassionate makes all the difference for me.

TROUBLESHOOTING: COMMON PROBLEMS

There are some common problems that you can look out for and that you can often nip in the bud if you spot them.

Forgetting to practise

'It just keeps slipping my mind.'

You've heard this before, I know, but not practising is probably one of the most common obstacles to progress. It's understandable because many people live busy lives while they are trying to change very well-established responses and behaviours. So it's not always easy to find the time and to get into the habit of practising regularly. However, here are things you can do to increase the chances of you remembering to practise:

- Try to fit it into your regular routine if you can. For example, link brief relaxation with waiting for your bath to run in the morning or getting into your car; or link practising your breathing with standing at the bus stop every morning.
- Use reminders – alarms in your mobile phone, sticky notes in key places at home – these will be your cues.
- Practise when you feel well as this is the ideal time to hone your skills – don't wait until you feel very anxious. It is all too easy to forget to practise when we are feeling OK.

Follow these guidelines and your skills will improve. You will find it easier and easier to use your coping strategies whenever you feel anxious and they will become part of your life.

Not catching anxiety early

'It comes on suddenly and I'm not prepared'

The key here is to routinely check your stress and anxiety levels – it is another habit you need to get into. In this way you can avoid being taken by surprise, you will 'catch' the early signs rather than being overwhelmed.

Giving up on a strategy too soon

'I want to feel better right away. This is taking too long – it's not working!'

It's human to want a quick fix, but learning new skills and new habits takes time. Not all the strategies in this book will be for you but before you abandon one of them think about why it might not be working. It could be because:

- You have not practised enough. The motto 'If at first you don't succeed, try, try again' is very apt.
- The technique and the situation are not well matched. Go through your range or list of strategies and give them all a try. Remember, distraction is not a good technique for tasks that require great concentration, such as driving, lengthy relaxation can only be used in certain situations and testing your thoughts is sometimes too difficult when you're on the spot, but can be done later.
- You tried the strategy when your stress levels were too high. Get familiar with the pattern of how your anxiety builds so you can catch it as early as possible. Any coping technique will work better if you are less stressed.

Self doubts

*'I don't think that I'll be able to manage my anxiety
for real.'*

Many people lack confidence in their ability to use their
new skills at first. It's understandable to ask questions like:
'What if it doesn't work?' and 'What if I get so wound up
that I forget what to do?' If you worry too much about
succeeding, it will be more difficult to manage your anxiety
so try to be open-minded about it. Try to have the attitude
that you'll just have a go and see what happens – however
it goes you'll learn more about your strengths and needs,
and you can adjust your subsequent practice accordingly.
If things don't go so well, you probably need to rehearse
your coping strategies a bit more. So, when you start to feel
those familiar worrying thoughts and feelings, think of it as
an opportunity to try out your new skills and to see what
happens: be curious rather than afraid.

*'I think I have a mixture of anxiety problems but my
doctor says it's generalized anxiety disorder. If I don't
know what I've got, how can I ever learn to cope?'*

It can be very helpful to understand what type of anxiety
problem you have – it can be reassuring to know that there's
a label for your experiences and that you are not alone. It
can also be helpful to know what the common maintaining cycles are for your anxiety. However, managing your
anxiety (whatever the label) will rely on you understanding just what makes *your experience* worse or better – and
you can use your anxiety diary to help you do this. When
you have a good sense of when you are most likely to be
feeling anxious, you can use your coping strategies to prepare yourself; when you are aware that your anxiety level

is rising, you can use them to keep it under control. So, whatever label or labels you have to describe your anxiety, managing it depends on understanding just when *you* need to use your coping methods.

'I'm OK in practice situations but I'll never manage in real life.'

It's normal to feel nervous when you're about to try something new and difficult. The beauty of having practised is that you'll have been honing your skills so that you stand a good chance of coping in real life. The best way is to start with something that you think you can take on now, and then gradually work your way up to the thing you most fear (see Chapter 10 on graded practice). Don't try to take on too much too soon as it could be off-putting and possibly disappointing. It's also important that you 'talk to yourself' in a gentle and encouraging way as you take on challenges. Try not to use the tone and vocabulary of a strict teacher as it might stress you out more.

'This is not going to be easy.'

This is quite true – in the short term – but in the longer term the challenge will become more manageable and you'll find it much easier to live without the anxieties and fears that currently undermine you. Although the idea behind managing your anxiety is quite simple and straightforward – learn to recognize it, catch it early and use a coping strategy that works for you – putting this into action is rarely quick and easy. At first it will be hard work as you keep detailed diaries, rehearse coping strategies, question your thoughts regularly and so on. However, once you have a better understanding of your fears and worries, and once you've mastered the techniques, you'll find it relatively easy to manage your problem.

GETTING A BALANCED LIFESTYLE

A final and very important tip for coping from now on is to get a balanced lifestyle. If you have struggled with anxiety for some time, then your life may have begun to revolve around it so you need to take a good look at how you spend your time and make sure that you are:

- *Developing relationships* as good friendships buffer us against all sorts of emotional problems.
- *Developing your interests and pleasures* so that fear and anxiety are not dominant in your life.
- *Getting active* as physical activity has been shown to improve mood and it's also a helpful distraction that burns off excess adrenaline and oxygen, which can otherwise make us feel physically uncomfortable.
- *Creating a good work/leisure balance*. Don't let work take over your life so much that your stress levels start to rise as this will make setbacks more likely.

LOOKING FORWARD

If you've read this book from cover to cover and practised the techniques you'll now have a number of strategies and some successes in coping with fear, worries and anxiety. Keep practising and you will consolidate your progress. It might be that you then go from strength to strength but we never know what life is going to throw at us and you might hit a difficult patch from time to time – it can happen to us all. If this happens to you, return to this book to refresh your knowledge and step up your practice so that you can refresh your skills. And always be compassionate with yourself when you hit troubled times. If you are still feeling anxious, despite having done these things, think about contacting some of the useful organizations at the back of this book. Remember that it's completely OK to ask for help and use available support around you. And don't forget that setbacks can be an opportunity to examine what went wrong and to refine your skills.

And finally: good luck!

USEFUL BOOKS AND RESOURCES

USEFUL ORGANIZATIONS

Mind
The leading mental health charity in England and Wales.
15–19 Broadway,
Stratford,
London E15 4BQ
Tel: 020 8519 2122 Fax: 020 8522 1725
Email: contact@mind.org.uk
Website: www.mind.org.uk

Anxiety UK
A website that targets searches for anxiety-related terms.
Website: www.anxietyuk.org

The Mental Health Foundation
Provides information and works to improve services for anyone
affected by mental health problems.
9th Floor,
Sea Containers House,
20 Upper Ground,
London SE1 9QB
Tel: 020 7803 1100 Fax: 020 7803 1111
Email: mhf@mhf.org.uk
Website: www.mentalhealth.org.uk

No Panic

Provides support for sufferers of panic attacks, phobias,
obsessive compulsive disorder and generalized anxiety disorder.
93 Brands Farm Way,
Telford, Shropshire TF3 2JQ
Tel: 01952 590005
(freephone helpline: 0808 808 0545, 10 a.m. – 10 p.m.)
Fax: 01952 270962
Email: ceo@nopanic.org.uk
Website: www.nopanic.org.uk

Triumph over Phobia UK

Helps sufferers of phobias, obsessive compulsive disorder and
other related anxiety problems.
PO Box 3760,
Bath BA2 3WY
Tel: 0845 600 9601
Email: info@triumphoverphobia.org.uk
Website: www.triumphoverphobia.com

First Steps to Freedom

Help sufferers of phobias, obsessive compulsive disorder, general
anxiety and panic attacks.
PO Box 476,
Newquay TR7 1WQ
Tel: 0845 120 2916
(freephone helpline 10 a.m. – 2 a.m.)
Email: first.steps@btconnect.com
Website: www.first-steps.org

British Association for Behavioural and Cognitive Psychotherapies

The organisation that regulates the practice of cognitive therapy
in the UK. If you are looking for professional support it is a
good idea to consult the BABCP website.
Imperial House,
Hornby Street, Bury BL9 5BN
Tel: 0161 705 4304 Fax: 0161 705 4306
Email: babcp@babcp.com
Website: www.babcp.com

USEFUL BOOKS

The Overcoming series, published by Robinson, includes many anxiety-related titles that are recommended on the NHS 'Books on Prescription' scheme. Subjects covered by the series include:

Overcoming Anxiety by Helen Kennerley
Overcoming Social Anxiety and Shyness by Gillian Butler
Overcoming Health Anxiety by David Veale and Rob Willson
Overcoming Obsessive Compulsive Disorder by David Veale and Rob Willson
Overcoming Worry by Mark Freeston and Kevin Meares
Overcoming Depression by Paul Gilbert
Overcoming Insomnia and Sleep Problems by Colin Espie
Overcoming Traumatic Stress by Claudia Herbert and Ann Wetmore
Overcoming Anger and Irritability by William Davies
Overcoming Panic and Agoraphobia by Derrick Silove and Vijaya Manicavasagar
Overcoming Low Self-Esteem by Melanie Fennell

Although the range of books listed above cover most bases, you might also find these self-help books useful:

The Compassionate Mind by Paul Gilbert, Constable
The Worry Cure by Robert L. Leahy, Piatkus
Mind Over Mood by Christine Padesky and Dennis Greenberger, Guilford Press
Assert Yourself by Gael Lindenfield, Thorsons
A Woman in Your Own Right: Assertiveness and You by Anne Dickson and Kate Charlesworth, Quartet Books

INDEX

Diary 1

When you feel anxious or scared or stressed, note what you do and how well it works for you.

Rate your levels of distress on this scale:

| 0 | 1 | 2 | 3 | 4 | 5 |

Not at all scared or stressed

As scared, worried or stressed as I can imagine being

When this happened and where I was	How I felt (rating)	What I did to cope	How I felt immediately	How I felt later	What I have learnt

Diary 2

When you feel anxious or scared or stressed, note how you feel, what you do and how well it works for you.

Rate your levels of distress on this scale:

0	1	2	3	4	5

Not at all scared or stressed
Calm

As scared, worried or stressed as I can imagine being

When this happened and where I was	How I felt (rating)	What was happening in my body and my mind	What I did	How I felt (rating)	What I have learnt

Diary 3

When you feel anxious or scared or stressed, note what goes through your mind.

Rate your levels of distress on this scale:

0	1	2	3	4	5

Not at all scared or stressed
Calm

As scared, worried or stressed
as I can imagine being

When this happened and where I was	How I felt (rating)	What was going through my mind: thoughts & images	What I did	How I felt (rating)	What I have learnt

Diary 4

When you feel anxious or scared or stressed, note what goes through your mind and then do a reality check by filling in the diary below.

Rate your levels of distress on this scale:

0	1	2	3	4	5

Not at all scared or stressed
Calm

As scared, worried or stressed as I can imagine being

What went through my mind	Why does my thinking make sense?	What are the 'pros' of my thinking?	What are the 'cons' of my thinking?	What doesn't fit with my thinking?	What's the worst thing that could happen?	How would I cope if the worst thing did happen?	What have I learnt?

Relaxation Record

When you do your relaxation exercises, write down how you feel before and after and how well it works for you.

Rate your levels of tension on this scale:

0	1	2	3	4	5

Calm, relaxed

As tense as I can imagine

Type of exercise Where and when?	Rating before	Rating after	What I have learnt

BOOST YOUR CONFIDENCE

MELANIE FENNELL

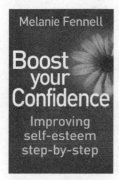

ISBN: 978-1-84901-400-7
Price: £7.99

Learn to recognize and embrace your strong points and stop low self-confidence in its tracks

Melanie Fennell has developed a similar, more accessible version of her bestselling book *Overcoming Low Self-Esteem*. Hugely readable and insightful, her CBT-based approach will help you to rebuild your self-confidence, step by step.

Poor self-confidence can affect many areas of your life, such as how you conduct your friendships and relationships and the extent to which you pursue your dreams and ambitions. Healthy self-confidence means being aware of your faults while at the same time recognizing your own personal strengths and talents. This invaluable book will help you to understand what knocked your natural self-confidence in the first place, what's keeping it down and how to start embracing your talents and strong points, enabling you to pursue the life you deserve.